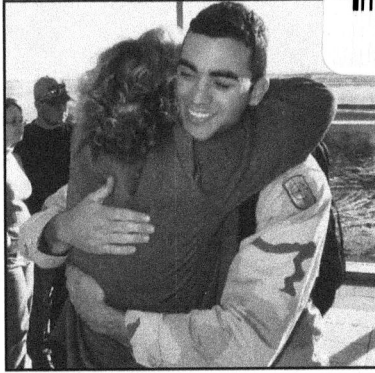

They Were Families

How War Comes Home

By Stephanie Mines, Ph.D.

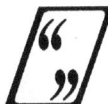

NEW FORUMS

NEW FORUMS PRESS INC.

Published in the United States of America
by New Forums Press, Inc.1018 S. Lewis St.
Stillwater, OK 74074
www.newforums.com

Library of Congress Cataloging-in-Publication Data Pending

This book may be ordered in bulk quantities at discount from New Forums Press, Inc., P.O. Box 876, Stillwater, OK 74076 [Federal I.D. No. 73 1123239]. Printed in the United States of America.

Photographs by Zach Street. Illustrations by Patricia Raine and Michele Stein.

ISBN 10: 1-58107-277-5
ISBN 13: 978-1-58107-277-8

"Prevention is better
than cure."

• Erasmus

Also by Stephanie Mines

Sexual Abuse/Sacred Wound:
Transforming Deep Trauma

We Are All in Shock:
How Overwhelming Experience Shatters You
...and What You Can Do About It

The Dreaming Child: How Children Can Help
Themselves Recover From Illness and Injury

New Frontiers in Sensory Integration

Contents

Dedication

This book is dedicated to OEF Veteran James Cody Green and his mother Sara Green. It is also dedicated to all the children of war, throughout all time and throughout the world.

Disclaimers

Nothing in this book is intended to substitute for consultation with medical professionals. Neither this nor any other book can replace the need for person-to-person medical attention. Please consult your physician for your medical needs. The resources in this book are designed to supplement and support your physician's recommendations.

To protect the privacy of many of the individuals whose experiences are conveyed in this book I have not used their real names. I have also altered the information about them sufficiently to make them unidentifiable. In some cases, however, individuals requested that I use their actual names.

Stephanie Mines, Ph.D.

Acknowledgements

Without the emotional, spiritual and practical help of others the unanswered cry for honorable services to the families of war might have broken me completely. My support team kept me going even as my own memories of how war came home to my family resurfaced.

I want to express my profound gratitude to Marian McGorrin who served as an outstanding editorial consultant, to Cynde Collins-Clark who I refer to in these pages as my chaplain, and to my student Michele Wilcox who rallied my spirits at moments of great sadness.

Zach Street graciously served as our photographer for volunteer models who helped to depict the applied touch interventions in Chapter Eight. This is my opportunity to let them know how much their generosity is appreciated. These visuals help significantly to transmit healing possibilities.

Finally I would like to thank the entire Board of Directors of Veterans Families United. They are my family in this mission.

Stephanie Mines, Ph.D.

Introduction

I was privileged enough to make contact with Stephanie Mines a few years ago. Our paths crossed because of our shared passion for supporting military and veterans' families.

I am an early years educator by background and have been part of a military family since 1991. My children and I have lived the life of a typical military family with frequent moves within the UK and overseas and long separations due to multiple deployments over my husband's career.

In 2009 I was asked by a school to visit a 5-year-old boy. His father had recently returned from a tour in Iraq and his mother was due to deploy to a non-conflict zone in two months. The boy had appeared to be coping reasonably well while his father was away but within a week of his father returning the school was extremely concerned about him. The child showed levels of significant aggression in class and used language that was far beyond his age. When I arrived in class I witnessed a very energetic child who was unable to stay still for even a second. His 6-year-old sister by contrast was quiet and very withdrawn. As a result of my observations, the school made an emergency referral to an Educational Psychologist who met the children within three days.

I was unforgettably struck by the manner in which the lives and learning of these children were shaped by how war had come home with their father. Unable to sit back and do nothing, these circumstances and my own experiences inspired me to set up my not-for-profit organization Service Children Support Network (SCSN) to offer support to children from military and veterans' families experiencing difficulties with transitions, separations and emotional wellbeing.

SCSN has three core purposes:
- To educate the educators so that they can better support the children in their care and to encourage parents to advocate for their children.
- To encourage research into this poorly researched area.

- To work directly with children in schools and the community and to advocate and support them.

Since 2009 we have served a wide range of children and their families. The concerns have been many and varied but are usually centred around frequent moves, separations and the additional needs that come from these stressors such as bereavement, trauma, mental and emotional health, special education and academic needs.

Frequent moves can be both positive and negative for children as they loose and gain friends and move in and out of different educational systems and schools. They have an opportunity to travel, often overseas, and this can give them a global perspective that their non-mobile peers may not have experienced. Deployment, however, has such an impact on families that I would struggle to think of any positives for the majority of children.

These children's stories often go untold. They cope with an enormous amount as a result of the context in which they live. I am surprised and disappointed by how often their needs are overlooked by service or agency providers. Indeed, I have sat open mouthed as policy makers and professionals have told me, "Children are not our priority."

Special educational needs can present a unique set of challenges to children who are part of the military community. In fact, some of my colleagues in the UK believe that military children with additional needs are the most vulnerable group of children within the military community.

Military parents and practitioners may not initially recognize special educational needs. Settling in to a new area is often seen as the reason for difficulties in the classroom. Conversely, sometimes children just need to reconnect and settle in a new environment but are too quickly labeled with an SEN (Special Education Needs) diagnosis.

Diagnosis is often a double-edge sword. No one wants to label children unnecessarily or use a deficit model but sometimes a label is needed to achieve recognition, finances and support. However, many military children never reach the diagnosis stage due to their mobile lifestyle. Like Stephanie, I too have seen parents' frustrations at being unable to secure consistent health or education services as a result of frequent relocations. Just like Justin's mother in Chapter Four they will often say, "We will be moving before that."

Despite these significant issues parents can step in and play a huge role in supporting their children. After all, they know their children better than anyone else. Parents should be encouraged and supported to act as advocates and practitioners should respect this knowledge and work with parents to gather their vital information. This knowledge can then be used to plan strategies, support and interventions both pastorally, and academically.

As Stephanie alerts us to in Chapter Four, military families may not be aware that support such as staying in one area is available. Even if they know about this support some military personnel may feel reluctant to ask for help fearing that it may seen as a weakness or impact on their career. Appropriate guidance at this juncture with a focus on the needs of children is absolutely vital.

On a personal level my husband was diagnosed with PTSD following a tour in the Middle East in 2005. I have spent over ten years searching for support and answers for my family to cope with this diagnosis and often struggled only to find neither. Stephanie offers clear information in a very accessible format. She gives the reader an insight into the issues faced by PTSD and polytrauma sufferers. She offers practical suggestions for family members left to pick up the pieces, as well as reminding us of the implications on the health and wellbeing of our families.

Stephanie's work gives readers the tools to use when supporting children. These tools will be useful for all children affected by war but also highly mobile children or children who experience separation from their parents or caregivers. I would encourage you to consider both traditional and innovative ways of supporting and advocating for your children or the children you teach or for whom you care. Advocacy is at the heart of Stephanie's work and therefore it speaks to me on both professional and personal levels.

This book would have been invaluable to me as I struggled to make sense of the world that had been turned upside down in my home. I have no doubt that this book will be an indispensible resource to anyone seeking to understand more about trauma and supporting families.

> Joy O'Neill FRSA, FHEA, MSc, Oxon,
> Founder Service Children Support Network,
> Visiting Fellow: Institute of Veterans and Families

Foreword

A reunion of veterans is a wonderful thing. I've attended reunions of World War II veterans for many years as a latter-day commander of the Army divisions they fought in, and observed their interactions. Then, in July of this year I attended a reunion of the rifle company I fought with in Vietnam. It was the first I've attended, and I had reservations about going. The vet who organizes the event each year said this is common.

I did not expect the emotional impact it had on me. These were men I had not seen in 45 years. As with the WWII reunions, I was struck with how many had been wounded. Some physical injuries were readily apparent – through prosthetic devices primarily. Some who appeared uninjured actually still retain bits of shrapnel in their bodies, and require periodic returns to the surgeon for repair. Then, of course, there were the emotional injuries that were not so apparent, unless the conversation veered in the proper direction.

So, years after the events, the trauma lingers. I hate to admit that as an Army officer serving for 37 years I have not been especially aware of the extent of this suffering. The impact of battlefield deaths is readily apparent, but for the wounded who were quickly evacuated my thoughts were often, "Good. He is only wounded and will get out of this danger and be OK from now on." Since I had not kept in touch with these comrades, I did not witness the ongoing tragedy in their lives.

Then, there were the family members attending the reunion. While my interaction with them was less frequent, I sensed from several discussions the strains on their family relationships as a result of combat experiences. Some of the vets had undergone more than one divorce, while others related how close they had come. I wondered how many of the children in these families had experienced emotional conflict. I thought, if I was impressed with the amount of suffering my fellow combat veterans experienced in those 45 years, how much greater had been the extent of the tragedy when their families were taken into account?

Stephanie Mines is on a mission. As the daughter of a World

War II infantry veteran, she personally experienced the tragic impact of posttraumatic stress disorder on a family. First in a previous title, and now in this excellent volume, I've witnessed her dedication and drive in addressing this little-known or understood problem in our society.

After completing the first title, *New Frontiers in Sensory Integration*, and early into the work on this book, we met for the first time during a gathering of an Oklahoma City support group for wounded veterans and their families. Notable during the meeting was her passion in addressing the problems discussed by those present.

Her work ranges widely and brings her into contact with a growing community struggling to address the issues explained in *They Were Families*. In the final stages of work on this title, she traveled to England, Scotland and Ireland, for example, where she conducted workshops and met families struggling with the same conflicts in those societies. She is untiring in her effort.

In this work, Dr. Mines strives to increase our understanding of the physiology of how war comes home and what we can do to end traumatic repetition in our time and so lessen its damages for future generations. Mercifully, she provides tools that can help us make a positive change in thousands of lives.

Today, only about one percent of the U.S. population serves in the military, and obviously an even smaller proportion experience actual combat. It is far too easy for our society to overlook the concerns of such a relatively small number, but of course the real question is, "How can we not do everything possible to help this select group of citizens who so uniquely served their country?"

This book is indeed part of a mission, and part of a grass-roots movement by families of veterans to address the catastrophic consequences when war comes home.

After the reunion with my Vietnam comrades, I struggled to define the unusual and pleasant emotion I felt, then finally one day I hit on the right word – healing. I hope this book provides that healing emotion for you, the reader!

> Douglas O. Dollar
> Publisher, Maj. Gen. (Ret.) USA

Overview

WHO IS THIS BOOK FOR AND HOW IS IT ORGANIZED?

A Note from the Author

"The key to healing is understanding how the human organism works."
☐ Bessel van der Kolk[1]

My purpose is to deliver into your hands and hearts the understanding of the physiology of how war comes home and what we can do to end traumatic repetition in our time and so lessen its damages for future generations. We are all the families of war. This said, I want you to know that this is a hopeful book; a book that assumes that people care and are willing to act on that caring. When we do not it is often because we do not know how. I wrote this book to change that.

They Were Families: How War Comes Home is divided into two sections. Section One: The Homeland of War provides insight, in easily understandable language, into the neurophysiology of war. The emphasis is on epigenetics, human development, and Secondary Traumatization. These are the phenomena that are center stage in the mechanisms of war coming home for adults and children. My purpose in this section is empowerment through education, awareness and understanding.

Section Two: Enlightened Home Strategies is the action component that follows directly from the learning in Section One. This is the resource bank for how family members, at home and without cost, can actively make a difference by stimulating health, listening compassionately and advocating for wellbeing.

These two sections are companions to improve the quality

of life for families inundated with the fallout that comes from violence, horror, terror and the overwhelming experiences that are coupled with combat and conflict. Above all else, children need to be protected from the intergenerational transmission of the ramifications of war. To provide that protection, adults need to recognize when and how that fallout happens. We must see our own Secondary Traumatization in order to identify it in someone else. When this is clear then an adult can be present for a child. Even a child's greatest suffering is ameliorated if someone stands for that child. You can be that someone.

Overview Note

1. Van der Kolk, B. (2014) The Body Keeps the Score: Brain, Mind, and Body in the Healing of Trauma. NY: Viking Penguin

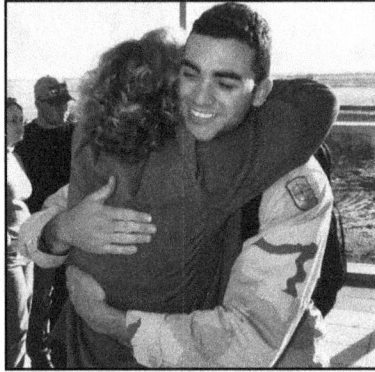

Section I
The Homeland
of War

Chapter One

The Mechanisms of Epigenetics and the Caregiver Steward

"Sometimes the greatest scientific breakthroughs happen because someone ignores the prevailing pessimism."
☐ Dr. Nessa Carey[1]

Sarah Landau was not herself a Holocaust survivor, but she lived her life as if that was her reality. She had chronic night terrors and panic attacks. She was hypervigilant and had an aversion to intimacy, very much like Naomi, her mother. Naomi was liberated from Auschwitz at the age of twelve. Fifteen years later she met and married her husband in New York, where Sarah was born, but Naomi never resolved her Holocaust experiences.

I became acquainted with Sarah when she interned with me during her graduate studies. She was preparing to become a psychologist and wanted to specialize in the treatment of trauma. Though at first she was reluctant to disclose much about herself, we eventually developed a good rapport. She said that it was never possible for her to bond with her mother because she was so secretive and withdrawn. Sarah was told only that her mother was in a concentration camp and that her mother's parents died there. When she was liberated, Sarah's mother was sent to live with distant relatives in the United States, the only ones left alive. Sarah knew little else about her mother's early life. She was tormented by how the mother she hardly knew seemed to inhabit her body and her life.

Sarah's answers lay in the mechanisms of epigenetics. The word means over, beyond or above genetics. It refers to external modifications of DNA that are caused by environmental impacts, such as environmental toxins. Research demonstrates that continuous emotional and psychological stressors can also be responsible for epigenetic impacts, and like other toxins, these can be transmitted to others. This means that how we interact with each other, and particularly how we interact with babies and young children who are highly receptive, sends neurochemical ripples that shape future generations for better, or sadly, for worse[2].

Epigenetics reveals how unvoiced emotional states shape genetic expression. In fact it is the studies of the offspring of Holocaust survivors, along with studies of babies born to mothers who were pregnant during the 9/11 terrorist attacks, that shed the most light on the mechanics of epigenetics[3]. Data reporting on the children of Vietnam War veterans also shows a statistically significant relationship between veterans' war experiences and their children's behavioral disturbances[4].

For epigenetic consequences to occur damaging influences must be repeated and impact development at key early thresholds. This differentiates these exposures from the Secondary Traumatization or Vicarious Retraumatization that are discussed in the next chapter.

The name for the process by which intergenerational transmission occurs is methylation. Exposure to trauma, including in-utero exposures, sufficiently changes hormonal states to create a shift that alters gene expression without altering genetic structure. When, how and with what frequency the exposure occurs determines the methylation or whether the impact turns certain immune system functions on or off. Persistent exposures are the most damaging. Genes are segments of DNA that contain instructions for activity. If gene expression is altered by persistent conditions then that alteration becomes transmissible as genetic material. It becomes heritable to the unborn. If, however, psychological damages can be interrupted before they become chronic repetitions, then traumatic repetition is also interrupted. That is what this book is about.

Epigenetics points us towards practical, viable and scientifically sound individuated interventions for trauma survivors and their offspring. In this chapter we explore what epigenetics tells us about how to protect and serve them.

Preventing Intergenerational Traumatic Repetition

"The application of epigenetic methods to the field of PTSD represents an exciting frontier because it gives us the ability to account for individual differences."
☐ Rachel Yehuda, Ph.D.[5]

There was no one in Sarah Landau's home to act as her advocate, or to protect her from the fallout of her mother's unresolved shock and trauma. If such an individual had stepped forward to assist Sarah in differentiating from her circumstances, her suffering would have been significantly less.

After her mother died Sarah eventually became that advocate for herself. She integrated what she learned as a trauma therapist and interacted with the fragmented younger part of herself to offer that child protection, safety and unconditional love. As a result of her determination to understand her epigenetic inheritance, Sarah guaranteed that the secondary traumatization that she had experienced would not be transmitted to her own children or to her children's children.

Sarah's path of self-observation, education and pro-active change teaches us what we, the adult stewards of children in the homes where war takes up residence, can do to prevent intergenerational traumatic repetition. These are the steps that Sarah took:

1. She identified the source of her nervous system fragmentation as being the byproduct of her mother's unresolved trauma;
2. She sought resources that would allow her to connect with early developmental stages in her life so that she could speak to them and differentiate them from the present;
3. She recognized her physiological sensations when she was activated as if the past were operative in the present;

4. She learned to engage with and eventually erase those sensations by providing new behavioral options for herself; and
5. She remained loyal to this practice of self-awareness so that
   eventually her nervous system recognized that there was a
   new safety in the present that had not existed in the past. Thus
   Sarah was able to fully inhabit the present.

Thanks to reports from people like Sarah who have inquired
into the mechanisms of epigenetics, including Nobel Prize winner
Eric Kandel, we can effectively end re-enactment[6]. When adults
do this for themselves, they recognize when children need this
support, and thus they can provide it for them in a child friendly
manner. How we are with each other changes our neurochemical
responses, and when positive interactions are repeated they also
make a definitive epigenetic impact.

If any one of us who has experienced trauma investigates
it and differentiates from it, that is a stand for ending traumatic
repetition. This is what I and others, like David Morris, author
of *The Evil Hours*, have done[7]. Readers can choose to follow our
model. Cumulatively these stands make a difference for humanity
even if they do not make headlines.

Through differentiation we generate a neurochemistry of resilience we generate a neurochemistry of resilience whether we are
caregivers, veterans, parents or therapists. Bessel van der Kolk,
in *The Body Keeps the Score*, explains how PTSD changes brain
physiology and thus becomes a force for epigenetic transmission[8].
Epigenetics, in fact, explains precisely how and why soldiers
returning from war are seen as being entirely different from the
individuals who enlisted. They are physiologically changed and
thus their behavior is unfamiliar to those who knew them before.
Combat shock transfigures individuals in the same way that the
Holocaust did, that rape does, and that any overwhelming experience that shatters one's sense of self, of time, and of reality must
reshape us. These experiences make safety elusive. By learning about epigenetics and making the courageous choice not to
engage in traumatic repetition we build safety for ourselves and
our families.

Safety and Attachment
Through The Eyes of a Child

At the core of Sarah's inability to feel close to anyone was the absence of personal safety that, for her, began in utero. Sarah's mother Naomi felt that her Holocaust memories were too horrible to share with others. The reason she gave herself for her silence was that she did not want to burden others with degrading images. This is the same reasoning that has, for millennia, made most war survivors reserved and withdrawn. This choice, however, actually perpetuates suffering by transmitting it in the form of a vague, chilling and disturbing atmosphere that infiltrates; some would use the word "infects," others.

Sarah's innate innocence and vulnerability at birth evoked her mother's grief. Instead of joy, Naomi felt a sense of the irreparable loss of her own innocence. This made it impossible for her to welcome her daughter with warmth. The tenderness that is natural between mother and child evaporated in Naomi's reactivation and she retreated away from Sarah rather than reaching for her. Without an explanation for this shocking loss of connection, Sarah took on her mother's emotional state, perhaps out of her longing to be close to her, so that it became her physiology. Naomi did not see Sarah as a separate person. She saw her as an aspect of herself. If she had managed somehow to recognize this, seek help and to communicate her dilemma to her daughter, it would have lessened the child's burden. "How," you might well wonder, "could a mother convey to her baby that her grief was not her child's fault?"

The simple answer is that just as Sarah knew that her mother was in pain, so too could she comprehend an explanation for that pain. Her mother, given guidance, could have said either out loud or intentionally, "My grief is not yours. You are not responsible for these feelings though you are exposed to them. I love you for who you are and will try my best to resolve my feelings of suffering from my past. They are not yours. Be free of them."

Such an articulation, imbued with awareness of a child's implicit intelligence, is the stuff of safety. Safety resides in being seen, in the acknowledgement of one's sensitivity and individuated existence, and not only in protection from outward danger. Safety is an inner experience of being contained that can sustain you even when threat is present. We have seen this time and time again when a courageous individual stands in their truth in the midst of disaster. We know that the consciousness of a developing child has the capacity to comprehend intentional and emotional states. Scientific research documents what loving, attentive parents always knew[9].

No one in Sarah's world knew that epigenetics was possible, or that her mother was withholding her love for her daughter out of her own terror and traumatic reactivation. No one believed that a baby or a young child had the level of sensitivity to absorb her mother's pain. Neuroscience confirms that the developing brain responds to everything in its environment, particularly the state of mind and the state of heart of one's primary caregivers. This is the experience of attachment and it shapes a child's learning and social engagement. We, as the stewards of children, can engage proactively to assure that a child lives a fulfilling life and experiences healthy selfhood despite being exposed to trauma in their home environment[10].

Sarah's indomitable curiosity and relentless pursuit of how she had become confused with her mother's suffering demonstrates both the mechanics of epigenetics and how we can unravel ourselves from them. Her story teaches us that protection for children resides in our recognition of their intelligence. Sarah's quest to find out what she experienced in her early development suggests a new path of stewardship by seeing through the eyes of children. My own experience with the children of veterans is that if we ask them directly about what they feel they will tell us their truth. It is our job to listen, believe them and then act on what they tell us.

The child within Sarah spoke of her loneliness and longing to feel the warmth and protection of her mother and her loving presence. Sarah's father loved his family but he expressed this by working night and day to earn the living that sustained them. He died of a heart attack not long after Sarah's mother died of lung cancer. Sarah entered adulthood as an orphan haunted by memories she could not clearly identify, but she graduated from this entrapment by looking into the eyes of her childhood and legitimizing her early needs.

Sarah Landau is not unlike you or me. Her courage drove her past resistance and passivity. Despite feeling daunted by the challenge of solving the mystery of her life she motivated herself to inquire into the neurophysiology of trauma. Most noteworthy is that she sought options outside the box of what others told her and even of her studies. She asked questions. Her perseverance is the model that inspires and motivates others. As someone who has followed this path I can vouch for its rewards. We serve our children when we heal ourselves.

The children of war are usually without one and sometimes both of their parents for periods of time. These separations have unavoidable developmental impacts. Military service, particularly combat, is life altering. Each deployment changes the soldier profoundly. When that soldier returns home he or she is not the person who left. If that soldier is a parent, these conditions, even without any additional details, will likely impact their child's attachment.

A soldier returning from the military theater is, under most circumstances, not in a good position to parent. The parent who was absent during military service is frequently absent in a different way upon return. Ruscio, et al., in a 2002 study, identified avoidance and emotional numbing as the primary culprits[11]. From a child's point of view, when a parent acts out unresolved trauma or cannot tolerate the stimulation of normal civilian life, or is unavailable, as Sarah's mother was, the environment is unsafe.

In a 2001 study of the children of fifty veterans of the War in Vietnam, Davidson and Mellor found that veterans exhibited a severe impairment of their ability to sustain a positive parent-child relationship[12]. The authors suggest that under almost all circumstances, depending on variables such as the magnitude of PTSD, the number of deployments and the nature of combat, the returning soldier is not in a position to engage in the normal interaction required to foster a meaningful and developmentally appropriate relationship with a child.

At least one adult in the household or in the family system

has to be designated as an advocate for the children of veterans. Without safe, secure attachment, children cannot learn and grow optimally. They will likely still progress in some ways, but usually at great expense to themselves, their families, and society as a whole.

Sarah Landau played catch-up when she became her own advocate as an adult. We can save children from that prolonged struggle and assure that they enjoy the learning and freedom of childhood by recognizing what it means to be their stewards when they are young. If we know, for instance, that a child experienced early trauma that preceded the conditions that war brings home, we can posit that they will be more vulnerable to retraumatization.

This discussion is part of an evolving definition of what it means to be an actively advocating, engaged family member when war comes home. I would like to propose a new category of caregiving that I call Caregiver Stewards. Caregiver Stewards make an epigenetic difference in the outcomes for children and families.

What Does It Mean to Become a Caregiver Steward?

Both warriors and caregivers make sacrifices for something beyond themselves. The warrior does this on the battlefield; the caregiver does it at home. There are dangers in both arenas. It might appear that the caregiver has the easier and less risky assignment and certainly by some standards this is so. Nonetheless the caregiver faces challenges of the soul, of creativity, and crucial decision making. The caregiver's choices, like the soldier's, shape the lives of many others. Caregivers, like warriors, stand in the face of fire to deliver freedom, hope, and resources to those who are in need and vulnerable: the children of veterans and the children of war. The caregiver is at risk of infection from the contaminants of war. The nature of this risk and how to protect against it is described here and in the following chapter. The consequences of caregiving are real and impact health, quality of life and longevity. Our warriors today get short shrift and this causes them unforeseen pain, but their caregivers at home receive even less recognition and virtually no compensation.

Caregiver Stewards learn to cultivate the arts of pure listening and patience. They are students of a special brand of empathy that I call Resilient Empathy. This is empathy that acknowledges that evil occurs and that humans have to go through a process of recovery from exposure to it. Resilient Empathy also calls for self-empathy in setting personal boundaries. It is a preventative against Secondary Traumatization and is described further in that context in the next chapter.

Caregiver Stewards are required by their circumstances to embody these skills while simultaneously providing very practical services that maintain health and financial stability. In regard to children, this means assuring daily structures, a safe environment, nourishing meals, hearty play, consistent encouragement and secure attachment. This is a tall order that no one in Sarah Landau's home could fill. Sarah, however, because of her healing, made it her job as a therapist to assure that other children who needed a Caregiver Steward would have one.

How the Caregiver Steward Makes an Epigenetic Difference

"The terms 'taking care' and 'caring' imply cultivation of the person and the relationship."
☐ Dr. Arthur Kleinman[13]

Just as physicians and surgeons are saving the lives of wounded warriors with miraculous medical interventions, so are family members at home saving the lives and souls of their loved ones with their presence and caregiving. Most caregivers are likely unaware of their epigenetic power. Knowing the neurochemistry of true caregiving infuses it with joy and optimism. This neurochemistry is palpable and instrumental for the care of children.

The Neurochemistry of Love

Melinda's son Abe was bitter and broken. He had a Traumatic Brain Injury (TBI) and one side of his face had been burned almost beyond recognition. The remarkable plastic surgery he had endured did not change the fact that he was still permanently

11

disfigured. He bore little resemblance to the handsome young man who had enlisted. Abe's girlfriend could not handle it. She left him and went as far away as she could to avoid ever having to see him again. Abe, who had enlisted with such clarity and confidence, no longer knew what to do with his life. Everything that was familiar and meaningful to him was gone, except his family.

Melinda lost years of working income to be with her son during his surgeries. She was a licensed counselor but nothing had prepared her for this. She felt reduced to only one singular, reliable certainty: she would stand by her son. Her husband and daughter, Abe's older sister, agreed. They called themselves Team Abe and they shared a vow to do everything in their power to find resources and deliver them to their wounded warrior.

Team Abe bore witness to Abe. They honored Abe's journey and continued to relentlessly believe in him no matter how bad it got, including a long period when Abe lived behind a wall of silence, barricaded in his room. Melinda knew about setting boundaries. She created respite for herself and informed the other Team Abe members to do the same. She cultivated a support network and would let no one, including herself, sacrifice their own joy and wellbeing beyond what was healthy. No one in this network was wealthy, and coordinating compensations was a bureaucratic mess, but they shared the burden. They created spaces around them for decompression and they did their best not to over-extend so that they could truly bear witness to Abe.

It is impossible to remove a mother's pain at her son's disfigurement and apparent loss of potential, or a sister's grief, or a father's heartache. Mourning was a component of daily life for Team Abe. Nevertheless they generated enough collective love to build a force field of caring. This force field sustained them and ultimately it changed Abe's motivational responses sufficiently to allow him to turn the corner on his despair. Throughout his recovery Abe was silently steeping in survivor's guilt, resentment, horrific nightmares and excruciating physical pain. Though he punished himself relentlessly, he was not abusive to others. If he had been this story would be quite different. My article on domestic violence in military families along with my own experiential reports of my family life document this aspect of how war comes home[14]. Abuse and domestic violence require a different set of responses than Melinda's enduring patience, fortitude and networking. Abe's TBI was mild. If it had been more severe the remarkable outcomes this family finally realized would have been more difficult and would have taken much longer to attain. They might even have been impossible. Please see the chapter on TBI for additional information on addressing this signature wound.

It took years but Abe found a route to accepting himself as he was. He re-entered life; he let go of his resentment and his guilt and stepped into the present. He was grateful to be alive. To Abe's own amazement he is now the father of a beautiful son and a spunky daughter, and their lives fill him with beatific appreciation every day. His wife thinks he is a hunk and is proud of him. Abe learned how to compensate for his head injury. He attended TBI support groups and had the help of an excellent Occupational Therapist and other rehabilitation specialists who directed him brilliantly towards strategies to optimize his brain bank and to identify and compensate for his losses in memory and focus when they occurred. He learned to organize his life to avoid rekindling his head injury. He built a home based business and created structures so that he could manage his own time. His wife, with Melinda's help and the support groups they attended together, also educated herself about the wounds of war, including TBI, so that she could help monitor Abe's lifestyle and keep him in balance. Needless to say, with two children and two working parents this is not easy and they are not always successful, but Abe and his family feel whole now. Thanks to the enlightened Caregiver Stewards in Abe's family, his children are immunized against traumatic repetition.

Oxytocin, the neurohormone produced in response to empathic connection, and dopamine that surges when we become creatively immersed in problem solving, are two of the major ingredients in the neurochemistry of love. You may be surprised to know that curiosity also launches the oxytocin-dopamine formula, providing the primary ingredients for motivation. This chemistry is what allowed Sarah Landau, the remarkable woman you met at the beginning of this chapter, to overcome the depressive aspects of her history. Vigorous physical exercise, creative expression, prayer, meditation, being in nature, or anything that stimulates positive focus and excitement about overcoming obstacles, will also do it. The brain thrives on the lubrication of optimism, faith and belief. The neurochemistry of love introduces resilience into one's lineage.

Abe's story portrays the ramifications of recovery and transition when there is a Caregiver Steward on board. All the lessons were hard won. There were no quick fixes. Ultimately, though, Melinda modeled the Caregiver Steward by caring for herself while she was on the steep learning curve to support her son. Then she taught others in her family to do the same. Eventually Abe became his own Caregiver Steward just as Sarah Landau became her own advocate.

The Caregiver Steward's Creed

Caregiver Stewards, like Marines, honor a creed that informs all their actions, but particularly their actions under stress, when they are in harm's way, which for Caregiver Stewards is when they are utterly exhausted. I developed two aspects of a creed for Caregiver Stewards. The first is based on the Marine Creed and is a statement of priorities. The second itemizes what is required to maintain those priorities.

The Caregiver Steward's Creed

This is my body and my intelligence; my soul and my heart. They are my best friends and I must be mindful of them.

What counts are not how many hours I work but the quality of my presence.

What matters is my ability to optimize human potential for myself and for those in my care.

What I give is human service. Only humans can provide it. There is no machine, no drug, no system or agency that can offer what I provide.

Because this is so I will ever guard my human service from the ravages of disrespect, exhaustion and carelessness.

I will keep myself rested and regenerated, in body and soul.

Before God I swear this creed. Caregiver Stewards are the masters of compassionate, effective service for wounded warriors, families, and children. We are the guardians of recovery from the wounds of war, visible and invisible.

So be it, until all wars end and there is no longer a need for us.

The following list suggests the kinds of promises Caregiver Stewards make to themselves in order to fulfill their mission. While this list could certainly be longer, I hope I have managed to identify the central components, the "vows" you might say, that we caregivers need to take in order to, as the creed says, "guard" against depletion of our precious resources.

1. Recognizing that my primary instruments of caregiving are my intelligence and my health, I vow to protect these against depletion or disrespect;

2. I vow to utilize every resource available to sustain my caring presence, kindness, compassion and attunement to the ones for whom I am responsible;

3. Advocacy, including the right to know everything about a condition, asking pertinent questions, seeking second and third opinions, and researching options are my rightful actions as a Caregiver Steward;

4. I will honor my insights and awareness of what is needed based on my experience of those in my care;

5. Respite is my right and I will arrange it regularly for myself and others on my caregiving team to offset any possibility of exhaustion;

6. Networks of support will always be in place so that my caregiving is never the only available resource;

7. Identified resources and options for care will be posted in an obvious place so that others will have access to them;

8. I and my team members will create clear routines of care to prevent overwhelm and chaos;

9. I will not allow myself to become homebound and isolated;

10. I will not sacrifice my personal delights such as exercise, creative expression, reading, prayer, meditation, social outings or friendships;

11. I will ask for help as soon as I need it;

12. I will participate in a support group or another collective that allows me to debrief my experiences of caregiving;

13. I will stay abreast of new developments in healthcare and caregiving;

14. I will receive as much as I give; and

15. I will appreciate and honor myself for what I do.

The greatest gift a Caregiver Steward provides is clear, loving presence; being in the moment. Even though a Caregiver Steward is in the service of others, the primary loyalty is actually to themselves because they are the vehicles of caregiving. This requires attention to the symptoms of compassion fatigue. See the next chapter for resources to address compassion fatigue. Also see Chapters Seven and Eight to explore new avenues of regeneration.

When you honor the intent behind this creed you lessen the likelihood of Secondary Traumatization and epigenetic traumatic transmisson. All caregivers deserve to know that this is possible.

Chapter 1 Notes

1. Carey, N. (2011) *The Epigenetics Revolution: How Modern Biology is Reinventing our Understanding of Genetic Disease and Inheritance.* UK: Icon Books Ltd.

2. Yehuda, R., Daskalakis, N.P., Lehrner, A., et al (2014) 'Influences of maternal and paternal PTSD on epigenetic regulation of glucocorticoid receptor gene in Holocaust survivor offspring'. *American Journal of Psychiatry Aug; 171(8): 872-880.*

3. Yehuda, R., Cai, G., Golier, J.A., et al (2009) 'Gene expression patterns associated with PTSD following exposures to World Trade Center attacks'. *Biol Psychiatry* Oct; 66(7) 708-711.

4. Rosenheck, R., Fontana, A. (1998) 'Transgenerational effects of abusive violence on the children of Vietnam combat veterans'. *Journal of Traumatic Stress* Oct; 11(4):731-742.

5. Yehuda, R., Bierer, L.M. (2009) 'The relevance of epigenetics to PTSD: Implications for the DSM-V'. *Journal of Traumatic Stress* Oct; 22(5):427-434

6. Kandel, E.R. (2006) *In Search of Memory: The Emergence of a New Science of Mind.* USA: WW Norton & Co.

7. Morris, D.J. (2015) *The Evil Hours: A Biography of Post-Traumatic Disorder.* New York: Houghton Mifflin Harcourt. Mr. Morris' explorations of his experiences of PTSD from his exposures to trauma in Iraq have resulted in what are likely the most thoroughgoing insights into our current quagmire regarding the treatment of combat shock.

8. Van der Kolk, B. (2014) *The Body Keeps the Score: Brain, Mind, and Body in the Healing of Trauma.* USA: Viking Penguin.

9. DiPietro, J.A. (2004) 'The Role of Prenatal Maternal Stress in Child Development'. *American Psychological Society; 13*(2): 71-74.

DiPietro, JA. (2013) 'Fetal exposures to excessive stress hormones in the womb lead to adult mood disorders'. *Science Daily*, April.

10. Research into attachment is an ongoing investigation that was launched dominantly in the 1950s and '60s, most prominently in the work of John Bowlby and Mary Ainsworth. These more current references continue the quest to help parents and therapists comprehend this central theme in development. Recently parent groups have sprung up on social media and offer lively dialogues about their observations and experiences regarding attachment.

Schore, A.N. (1994) *Affect Regulation and the Origin of the Self: The Neurobiology of Emotional Development.* New Jersey: Laurence Erlbaum Associates Inc.

Schore, A.N. (2001) 'Effects of a Secure Attachment Relationship on Right Brain Development, Affect Regulation, and Infant Mental Health'. *Infant Mental Health Journal; 22*(1-2) 7-66.

Schuengel, C., et al. (2009) 'Children with disrupted attachment histories: Interventions and psychophysiological indices of effects'. *Child and Adult Psychiatry and Mental Health; 3*:26

Fegert, J.M., Ziegenhain, U. (2009) 'Early intervention: Bridging the gap between practice and academia'. *Child and Adult Psychiatry and Mental Health; 3*:23.

11. Ruscio, AM., et al. (2002) 'Male War Zone Veterans' Perceived Relationship with their Children: The Importance of Emotional Numbing'. *Journal of Traumatic Stress Oct; 15*(5) 351-357.

12. Davidson, AC., Mellor, DJ. (2001) 'The adjustment of Australian Vietnam veterans: Is there evidence for the transmission of the effects of war-related trauma?'. Australian-*New Zealand Journal of Psychiatry* Jun; 35(3) 345-351.

13. Dr. Arthur Kleinman is the author of numerous books that develop an understanding of the caregiving dynamic. He is a physician and a medical

anthropologist. His writings include *The Illness Narratives, The Social Origins of Distress and Disease,* and countless articles and blogs on the experiences of giving and receiving healthcare.

14. Mines, S. (2007) 'Domestic Violence Within Military Families'. *Encyclopedia of Domestic Violence*, NY, Routledge; 487-492

Chapter Two

Transcending Secondary Traumatization

Protective Strategies for the Families of Veterans and Combat Shock Survivors

"How can someone who is holding so many traumas be of service to someone else if they are full up? You've got to empty the glass."
☐ Mariska Hargitay[1]

We can actively prevent the intergenerational transmission of trauma in our families. Shelby Garcia who was nine years old when her father returned from Iraq with undiagnosed PTSD and an undetected Traumatic Brain Injury says, "My family should have been educated about these conditions before my father came home, not years later, after the damage was done. By the time we found the therapy we needed for our family we had already been through bankruptcy, my brother and I had both experienced major meltdowns, and my parents were in crisis."[2]

Shelby is now in graduate school studying to become a counselor in order to serve the children of military families. She encourages me with her determination, insight, perseverance and compassion. She knows that by addressing the impacts of war on children we simultaneously transcend Secondary Traumatization and prevent epigenetic replications. She is acting on that understanding to make a difference in the world.

Joy O'Neill, who wrote the Introduction to this book, is a military wife and parent. She is also an educator and a service children's advocate. Joy alchemized her exposures to Secondary Traumatization into creating the Service Children Support Network in Britain.[3] After witnessing how the special needs of the children of military families go unanswered time and again in the educational system, and after seeing what happened to her own three children when war came into her home, Joy could not remain passive. She had to take the next step and become a voice for service children. She is relentless in her mission to represent service children worldwide. Shelby and Joy provide me with abundant hope that we will turn this corner on a centuries old neglect of military families and finally fulfill our obligations to them.

This chapter supplies education about Secondary Traumatization that is designed to heighten your awareness of its onset along with the tools to transcend it. The hands-on supports you need to interrupt Secondary Traumatization in your nervous system can be found in Chapter Eight. If, as you learn about Secondary Traumatization and find your unique route to its transcendence, you should decide to join Joy, Shelby and me in becoming a voice for military children, we welcome you into our ranks.

What is Secondary Traumatization?

Arguably everyone in contemporary society is suffering from some degree of Secondary Traumatization as a result of incessant exposures to violence via the media and global sensory overload. My book *We Are All in Shock* is about these phenomena. *We Are All in Shock* gives a broad overview of the physiology of overwhelming experience, beginning early in life, and how the human nervous system can be repaired and regenerated.[4] What the families of veterans experience is of an even higher order of magnitude because our Secondary Traumatization is cultivated daily by exposures to the physical, psychological and moral distress of someone we love.

An analogy for comprehending Secondary Traumatization is to see that it operates neurologically just as infection or contamination operates in the immune system. We absorb trauma through the stress hormones we interact with and also utilize while engaging and living with someone who is traumatized. Just as we become ill when we are in the same place where bacteria or a virus are active, so do we become traumatized when our lives are thrown permanently off track because of the needs and behaviors of a traumatized individual. Another analogy is that the impacts of Secondary Traumatization resemble what happens when non-smokers breathe second hand smoke. This causes the same kind of cancer that kills smokers. Similarly those who care for the severely traumatized inhale PTSD symptoms despite not having witnessed or endured the traumatizing events directly. This transference of maladies is so common that the characteristics can be itemized. They include, but are not limited to:

1. Dejection;
2. Confusion;
3. Memory loss;
4. Insomnia;
5. Nightmares;
6. Intrusive horrific imagery;
7. Guilt;
8. Loneliness;
9. Dissociation;
10. Fatigue;
11. Hyperarousal;
12. Hypersensitivity;
13. Irritability;
14. Headaches; and
15. Anxiety.

Most striking is how Secondary Traumatization robs family members of optimism. When this occurs then the situation is critical. The individual needs help immediately. If a family member no longer appreciates what they previously enjoyed, if their entire sense of self becomes that of someone who is deeply and chronically unhappy, then the degree of Secondary Traumatization is severe. Throughout this book you find a variety of resources for regeneration from Secondary Traumatization. Use them! These resources, along with becoming educated about Secondary Traumatization and how it operates, are essential to its transcendence. The symptoms of Secondary Traumatization will not go away unless you act. Untreated Secondary Traumatization eventually becomes heritable, You can effectively engage and actively prevent that outcome.

The Physiology of Secondary Traumatization

If we know how something happens, we can undo it. We are alive in a time when the mysteries of the human body and its functions are revealed more and more every day. This is incredibly empowering. We are, nonetheless, required to be self-directed and to invest our time and attention to take advantage of these revelations. This investment is one that is guaranteed to give returns. It is the key that unlocks the gateway to health. It is the path to self-advocacy that has been shown to make a real difference in health outcomes.[5]

When veterans return from theaters of war their unprocessed trauma comes home with them. They are given little if any time to debrief their horrific experiences before being sent back to civilian life. Families, therefore, receive the first raw, unfiltered download, even when nothing is said. Veterans themselves are unconscious of the magnitude of unprocessed trauma they embody. In the midst of combat and in military life there is no time for this sorting. Indeed, it is discouraged. Life depends on hypervigilance. It is only when threat is no longer a constant that the underbelly of trauma and shock is exposed like a beached whale. Survivors are flooded by disorganized, chaotic and hightened physiological sensations over which they have no control. The masters of war never prepared them for this onslaught. Because families are generally so eager to welcome their veteran home, they welcome, all too readily, the untold stories that linger in the soldier's field and that have rearranged his or her identity.

Therapists and care providers train themselves to create boundaries, detachment and distance from these unresolved, contaminating issues. These protections are much less available to family members. On the contrary, they may be completely unnatural to them. To be prepared for the return of veterans from combat zones an entirely different stance is required for family members; one that they must consciously learn. It is called Bearing Witness. If family members combine Resilient Empathy with Bearing Witness they will have hopeful allies to avert Secondary Traumatization and serve combat survivors with less damage to themselves.

The Difference Between Epigenetics and Secondary Traumatization and Why Early Intervention Matters

Epigenetics reveals how chronic exposures to environmental contaminants, including toxic emotions and psychological influences, as well as substantive toxins like lead or smoke, modify gene expression. These are not actual changes in DNA. Rather they are changes in DNA sequencing caused by chemical lags that are known as methylation. Secondary Traumatization, on the other hand, is a stress response that results from the levels of exposures to trauma that occur for people who help a traumatized individual or a group of trauma survivors over a period of time. The stress hormones that result from Secondary Traumatization, if unrelieved, lead to an epigenetic impact. This is precisely why early recognition, respite and regeneration are critical. The sooner that Secondary Traumatization is identified and treated, the less likely that health consequences and epigenetic transmission will follow. Other terms that have been used for Secondary Traumatization are Compassion Fatigue and Vicarious Retraumatization or Vicarious Traumatization.

When Shelby Garcia, the inspirational young woman I mentioned earlier in this chapter, decided to put boundaries around her relationships with her traumatized parents, she assured that her stress response would not become epigenetic. As a nine year old, Shelby was overwhelmed by concern for her parents whose struggles, arguments and distress she saw every day of her young life. She stepped into the role of being their mediator. This was inappropriate for her age and did not meet her developmental needs, but it is what this remarkable person did to survive and to express her love. Shelby has specifically asked that her real name be used in this book. She does not want to mask her discoveries. She wants to honor them. When Shelby learned about Secondary Traumatization and saw, many years later, what she had done in response to it, she could choose to stop playing the role of the family mediator. She did not know she had this option earlier. When she discovered it, she made a swift decision. She became herself. She terminated the Secondary Traumatization exposures for herself and future generations by stepping out of the mediator role.

Like Sarah Landau in Chapter One, Shelby had to voluntarily educate herself as an adult about Secondary Traumatization and epigenetics. Sarah's exposures began in utero, making epigenetics a reality for her. Shelby, on the other hand, experienced a relatively well attached early life. Her first experience of Secondary Traumatization occurred when her father deployed to Iraq and her family life went topsy-turvy. Conditions worsened with every subsequent deployment and became explosive after her dad returned home from his final term of service. Knowing this now, Shelby is already well qualified to advocate for military children.

I have experienced Secondary Traumatization not only because of growing up in a war torn home, but as a result of writing this book. When I recognized the magnitude of damage to military families worldwide from the universal failure to care for them properly, I felt drained and disempowered. The despair was palpable to me, and I could feel how it could lead to depression. I was as if possessed by the ghosts of neglected military children and families. This reactivation stole my enthusiasm and creativity in a way that alarmed me. I relived the abandonment I felt as a child when there was no adult available to protect me from how my father was when he returned from combat. I became enraged, yet my rage seemed futile, just as the rage of military families abandoned by a lack of adequate or appropriate services often feels futile.

I faced these obstacles and dealt with them using resources that I offer in this book, but it took more effort than I could predict. The fact that military family dilemmas such as those I share with you persist for so long, and the fact that these dilemmas are so thoroughly ignored by social and governmental agencies worldwide makes the burden heavy. Nevertheless, in the same way that I fought back as a child to not be defined by my father's violence, so do I now fight back to not be silenced in writing and releasing this book. This represents an ongoing process of defending against Secondary Traumatization, rather like building immunity against disease. It has two major aspects:

1. Itemizing and emphasizing victories; and
2. Recognizing and inviting collaboration.

When I recall that I actually triumphed over my circumstances and that I am not alone, I am invigorated. Feelings of defeat, despair and loss are consumed by a sense of possibility. I have to name the unity, for instance, that I feel with Shelby Garcia. She and I navigated the undiagnosed TBI coupled with PTSD in our fathers when they returned from war. Shelby and I are linked in our crusade for education, advocacy and prevention. Because we are linked, we are surely part of a larger movement. This helps me acknowledge that there are surely others who are working alongside me to end this cycle. This encourages me to recognize the difference between now, when I have colleagues, and earlier, when I felt stranded and isolated.

When I see that I am the victor over conditions that do not ultimately define me and that I am a voice for change, I claim my empowered identity. Through these recognitions and a deeper commitment to the truth of who I am I fight off the virus of Secondary Traumatization and regain my health and my energy. This is my path of individuation and differentiation. I offer it as a model. It is vitalizing, energizing and motivating. I repeat it frequently and I am here to share it with you.

I was reactivated in writing this book because epigenetics have marked me, and like Sarah Landau, they are part of my inheritance. Whenever someone has a history of very early trauma, especially in utero, and when trauma is a component of their family lineage, Secondary Traumatization is more likely. Nevertheless my efforts to educate myself and the awareness that I have cultivated prevents the transmission of this history to my children and to my grandchildren.

In the pages of this book I speak to you about resolving Secondary Traumatization not just as a clinician but from my experience with the heart of this disease. I have cultivated a force that is stronger than the repeated dictums like: "Do not speak. Do not talk about this. Do anything else but talk about how war comes home. Eat, drink, watch a movie, turn on your computer, go to sleep, do anything rather than name the elephant that lives in your house." I have silenced that repressive voice. When we speak out, seek help, and shake off Secondary Traumatization, we transcend it. If we remain silent, we perpetuate it.

In addition to Sarah Landau, Shelby Garcia and Joy O'Neill whom I have already mentioned, I want to introduce you to the remarkable Cynde Collins-Clark. Cynde is the mother of Operation Iraqi Freedom (OIF) Veteran Joe Collins, who continues to struggle in his recovery from PTSD, toxic exposures and other war and combat related conditions. Cynde partnered with me to create the REST House family centered transition design that you can review at the end of this book. She is the seed energy behind Veterans Families United, a nonprofit organization she developed to provide networks, guidance and inspiration for the families of veterans.[6] Sarah, Joy, Shelby, Cynde and I represent the mothers, the children, and the family members who are transcending Secondary Traumatization. We are not "studying" it for research purposes. We are transcending it for ourselves, for our families and for future generations. We live to make a difference in this cycle that must come to an end now.

What I extend to you regarding resolving Secondary Traumatization is not experimental. It is a living practice. The tools in this book are delivered by and to those who live day to day, hour by hour, with how war comes home. Shelby Garcia says, "I just needed someone to talk to," in reflecting back on what her nine year old self missed. In many cases, Secondary Traumatization lessens when someone listens. Often people can sort out their own needs if they are truly heard.

The contaminants of Secondary Traumatization are already in humanity's blood stream where they have been festering for years. This epidemic is surfacing so that it can be treated. The mask of avoidance is peeling off.

Bearing Witness and Resilient Empathy: The Twins that Guard Against Secondary Traumatization

Bearing Witness can be described as loving consciously, and loving while at the same time protecting one's own nervous system. It is the twin of Resilient Empathy. They both require intentionality and mindfulness. Neither implies withholding or limiting the love that one gives to another. Bearing Witness and Resilient Empathy are so symbiotic that sometimes they are indistinguishable from each other.

Bearing Witness is a stance; a way of seeing. It interacts and co-collaborates with Resilient Empathy. Both erect clear boundaries that allow us to differentiate self from other. Bearing Witness is the state of being and Resilient Empathy is cultivated through inner awareness to produce and project loving objectivity and neutrality. Both increase our capacity to be of service with some degree of equanimity and lessen vulnerability to Secondary Traumatization.[7]

Carl Rogers was perhaps the first theoretician to examine the healing nature of empathy which he defined as "temporarily living in the other's life." Rogers invoked empathy as a central aspect of the congruence he felt was critical for successful therapeutic dynamics. He said empathy meant "being with another in the way that means that for the time being you lay aside your own views and values in order to enter another's world without prejudice."[8]

What I am suggesting here is the harnessing of this heart based empathy and anchoring it with personal boundaries that imply empathy for oneself in the midst of overwhelming traumatic exposures. In this way one is not flooded by the needs of another. The person in a state of Resilient Empathy maintains a clear headed confidence in the healing process. Bearing Witness is seeing clearly without flinching and looking directly at the core truth, beneath appearances. The two together project warmth and strength.

If we are not mindful of our reception to how war comes home, we run the risk of circulating the same neurohormones that are associated with trauma, like cortisol. Excessive cortisol

27

production damages the immune system. The threat hormones that are produced by PTSD and Secondary Traumatization cannot sequence to completion. They cannot metabolize. They are stored in the body. The same applies to unsequenced adrenaline or epinephrine.

If family members are alert to these ramifications before transition occurs, prevention may be possible. When Secondary Traumatization is already active, individuation and differentiation can be rallied, consciously, as antidotes. I described how I went through that process while writing this book. It is never too late to recover. The best time is now.

How Do I Know If I Am In a State of Secondary Traumatization?

As mentioned earlier, to varying degrees everyone in modern society is in a state of Secondary Traumatization. We have normalized it. The conditions for the families, and especially the partners and children of veterans, are much more severe and therefore have greater physiological consequences. Children require the attention and therapies that are tailored for them. See the following chapter for guidance regarding Secondary Traumatization and children. Consider the questions that follow and if you answer them largely in the affirmative, this would suggest that you are in the grip of Secondary Traumatization. These questions apply for people of all ages.

1. Do I have difficulty enjoying the things I once enjoyed for myself and with others? This includes hobbies, exercise, outings and social gatherings.
2. Do I have difficulty unwinding and relaxing? Do I, for instance, stay anxious about my "to do list" for so long that I cannot sleep?
3. Do I generally feel anxious more often than not?
4. Do I have trouble falling asleep or sleeping through the night?
5. Do I experience disturbing and intrusive imagery that interferes with my ability to be present?

6. Am I often irritable, for instance with my children, friends or with co-workers or other family members?
7. Do I have frequent headaches and other unexplainable physiological discomfort?
8. Do I have lower back pain?
9. Do I have discomfort and pain between my shoulder blades?
10. Has my memory become worse?
11. Do I tend to lose things more often, such as my keys?
12. Do I sometimes feel numb, cynical or hardened?
13. Do I resent other people's happiness and joy?
14. Am I much more exhausted then I used to be?
15. Do I feel despair about the world?
16. Do I have difficulty believing in an optimistic future for myself or for humanity?
17. Do I feel isolated and alone in the world?
18. Do I avoid opportunities to share my experiences with others? Am I less sociable and generally more withdrawn?
19. Do I feel on the alert most of the time?
20. Do I find myself thinking about others, and especially the problems of others, more than I think about my own needs?

Transcending Secondary Traumatization

If you answered yes to most of these twenty questions, there are some actions that if taken immediately and consistently will relieve Secondary Traumatization. In the process, as a bonus, you may find that you also experience an upgrade in your understanding and behavior. This is how way resiliency works. Resiliency awakens new learning and spontaneity. It occurs naturally as you unravel Secondary Traumatization.

The formula for dispelling Secondary Traumatization consists of the following elements:

1. Individuation or differentiation from trauma or the traumatized individual. This does not mean turning your back on anyone. It means understanding and feeling, in your body, that you are an entirely unique individual. You empty absorbed feelings out of your individuated system and become full with who you are and with your awareness of the present moment. This is not an

act of selfishness. It is the opposite. Until you individuate you cannot truly connect with others as who you are.

2. Prioritizing yourself by engaging in what you may find enjoyable and enriching, such as journal writing, physical exercise and walks in nature, pleasurable hobbies, social engagements with those you trust and are comfortable with, and the most regenerative choice of all: rest. If rest seems illusive try attending a restorative yoga course or learn about prayer and contemplation. Ask for help. Make your needs essential because they are. You cannot meet the needs of others if yours go unmet.

3. Immune support using, for example, the applied touch remedies contained in this book; re-evaluating your diet to make it more supportive of immune function and perhaps seeking healthcare providers to advise you or investigating new dietary options. Taking time to care for yourself will automatically enhance the vitality of your immune system.

4. Self-assessment, like reviewing your history to see if there are self-sabotaging or destructive patterns at play. Journaling is a wonderful way to explore your feelings. Journaling is a wonderful way to self-asses. It can reveal what makes you vulnerable to Secondary Traumatization. See Chapter Seven for writing structures that can assist you with self-assessment.

5. Re-engage with the valiant part of yourself by remembering your triumphs and itemizing the times in your life when you overcame difficulties. Journaling is again an excellent way to do this.

Finally I want to suggest the role that faith can play as a possible antidote to Secondary Traumatization. I am not speaking of any specific faith, but of faith generally.

Chaplaincy

Cynde Collins-Clark, the Director of Veterans Families United (VFU), is a woman of faith. She opens and closes every VFU Board meeting with prayer. She regularly invites Board members to pray for each other. Cynde practices many forms of self-care such as taking regular personal retreats, spending time with her wonderful husband, receiving healing treatments, and dancing. But above all else Cynde's greatest resource as she tends to the needs of her veteran son, networks among agencies and ministers to the many families that turn to her for direction, is her faith. In this regard I see her as a chaplain, the one who invokes faith. To me she is the chaplain of her home and the chaplain of Veterans Families United. When I attend VFU Board meetings she is my chaplain. When I receive a memo from Cynde asking me to pray for a VFU Board member, I receive that request as coming from a chaplain.

What I mean here is not that Cynde is convincing me of any faith in particular but that she is reminding me of the role and power of faith. She is stimulating in me the awareness that I am not alone in what I do, and that there are not only others, but also that there is an energetic field with which I am aligned and which resonates with me and my efforts. Others in the healthcare field have commented on the beneficial impacts of faith in recovery from a broad spectrum of illnesses and research has documented this affect.[9] No matter what faith appeals to you, whether it is an organized practice or the choice to practice independently in your home or in the temple of the natural world, the cultivation of faith is one of the antidotes to Secondary Traumatization.

I recently heard a broadcast about a group of school children who were placed in a concentration camp in China during World War II. The imprisoned adults who were responsible for these children, all of whom were separated from their parents, chose to sustain practices for and with them that upheld their optimism and faith. The children were led in song, mostly hymns, and they were instructed to remain dignified, polite and clean under all circumstances, to the best of their ability. The adults kept the children engaged in learning and healthy play despite their horrible surroundings. Those who survived remember their concentration camp experience as a great teaching rather than as a trauma. The adults in the camp were their chaplains.

Will you be the chaplain of your family in the way that is appropriate to your environment? Can you invite the power of faith to transcend the forces of Secondary Traumatization? That faith does not even need a name. Faith of any kind can turn the tide of Secondary Traumatization when war comes home. Faith invites creativity and the neurological resiliency that is essential if we are to end traumatic repetition. Whatever your faith may be, become its chaplain and invoke its power.

Chapter 2 Notes.

1 Hargitay , M. Taken from "Vicarious Trauma" on the Joyful Heart Foundation website. The mission of the Joyful Heart Foundation is to heal, educate and empower survivors of sexual assault, domestic violence and child abuse, and to shed light into the darkness that surrounds these issues. JoyfulHeart was founded by Mariska Hargitay in 2004. www.joyfulheartfoundation.org.

2. 2015, June 22nd. Excerpt taken from Dr. Mines' personal interview with Shelby Garcia.

3. Joy O Neill is a teacher, researcher, and founder of The Service Children Support Network (SCSN), based in Buckinghanshire, England. SCSN is an independent, not-for-profit social enterprise that works in collaboration with the MOD (Military Office of Defense) and Military Welfare Organization to support educational and welfare professionals and members of the military in their roles in supporting Military Service children and their families. See the website: servicechildrensupportnetwork.co.uk

4. Mines, S. (2003) *We Are All In Shock: How Overwhelming Experiences Shatter You .... And What You Can Do About It.* NJ: The Career Press.

5. Self-advocacy in healthcare is a growing field of research. All signs point to improved health outcomes when individuals actively advocate for themselves by asking questions and doing their own investigative research. J. A. Jonikas, et al, (2011) for instance, found that mental health patients who self-advocate experience fewer psychiatric symptoms. R.A. Adams (2010) documents that when patients actively interact with their health care providers, their health outcomes improve. Research is also replete with studies that show that under-served populations are less likely to self-advocate because they are not prepared to do so, do not have access to information, or have not been educated about that possibility. This includes veterans and their families who deserve to be informed about how to self-advocate and their rights to do so.

6. Veterans' Families United Foundation; Resources for Friends and Families of Veterans. See the website: veteransfamiliesunited.org

7. Eres, R., Decety, J., Winnifred, R.L., Molenberghs, P. (2015) Individual differences in local gray matter density are associated with differences in affective and cognitive empathy. *NeuroImage.* Aug 15; 117: 305-310

8. Rogers, C.R. (1980) *A Way of Being.* 142-143. New York: Houghton Mifflin.

9. Dossey, L. (1993) *Healing Words: The Power of Prayer and the Practice of Medicine.* New York: Harper Collins. Newberg, A., D'Aquili, E., Rause, V. (2001) *Why God Won't Go Away: Brain Science and the Biology of Belief.* New York: Random House. Doidge, N. (2007) *The Brain that Changes Itself: Stories of Personal Triumph from the Frontiers of Brain Science.* New York: Viking Penguin. Feldman, David B. and Kravetz, Lee Daniel (2014), *Supersurvivors: The Surprising Link Between Suffering and Success.* New York: Harper Collins.

Chapter Three

In Our Children's Names: Advocating for the Children of War

"Trauma itself does not inevitably lead to anxious attachment or insecure attachment. It is possible for children to experience trauma and other hardships, but because their caregivers are adequately protective in response to the dangers, they will have secure or relatively secure attachment strategies."
☐ Chris Purnell, Ph.D.[1]

Eight year-old Michael kept burning things down. He started with the kitchen trash and moved on to the shed behind his house. That was when the authorities stepped in. Michael had counted the days until his father returned from Iraq. He had been disappointed so many times that he could hardly believe it would ever really happen. When it did, though, Michael was confused. The man sitting in the corner of the living room playing video games did not resemble his dad. Where was the father who played games with him, ruffled his hair, and took him on adventures? It had been so long since that father had lived with him that Michael wondered if maybe he had made him up. Maybe that father never existed. His mother grew sadder and quieter. This had been going on since his dad first deployed but now it was much worse. Michael heard them arguing at night and it scared him. Sometimes it sounded like things were crashing in the house, but Michael covered his ears and curled up in his bed and forced himself not to listen.

When the police came to the house to talk about the fires

Michael's mother was speechless. She looked at her son with disappointment and Michael felt immediately that he had let her down. He had made things worse. She never said that, but then his mother was saying less and less all the time. Later that night Michael heard his father shouting that what happened was his mother's fault. What had she taught his son while he was in Iraq? What had she done to make him this way?

Punishment was the first thing that Michael's father thought of, but it was the last thing that Michael needed. Everyone kept asking Michael "why", but he could never find the words to answer them. It was Michael's aunt who suggested therapy. She was watching her nephew slip away, losing the joy she remembered him having before, when the family was whole.

Children find their sense of safety and trust through their attachment to their parents. As a small child Michael had that healthy attachment, before his father went to Iraq. With each deployment it seemed that connection weakened incrementally and changed to anxious attachment.[2] As his mother also seemed to fade away, retreating regularly to her bedroom or working late, Michael felt stranded, though he would not have known how to express that feeling.

Michael was often left in the care of his older sister Deirdre who resented this responsibility and punished Michael in every way she could. She had lost what was once her reliable connection to her mother along with her father's attention. Once she was his "princess" but now it seemed he did not even remember her. Deirdre was in the throes of puberty and her anger became an underlying, smoldering constant. The entire family was burning up with a passionate need to be reunited and restored, but no one knew how to create that. Michael's natural need for attention drove him, instinctually and compulsively, to start fires. He was not doing this deliberately, of course. He was unconsciously sending out blazing, raging siren calls for help in the only way his body could find. Developmentally he was not yet capable of articulating his motives. His actions, despite their appearance, were innocent. In ways that are impossible to explain easily he was acting out the dilemma of everyone in his family.

Michael's dilemma is re-enacted over and over again in a variety of ways in the homes of military families. Every military child needs and deserves someone to be their advocate and to assure their sense of safety, optimism, hope, and enthusiasm. What Michael and Deirdre were burning for was someone who could be:

1. Present and caring;
2. Curious about them;
3. Co-participatory and developmentally attuned;
4. Interactive and synchronous with them;
5. Consistent; and
6. Connected.

When Michael's aunt and uncle consulted with me about the situation in Michael's home, I gasped. Michael was doing exactly what my brother had done when our father came home from war sixty years ago: setting buildings aflame. Michael's aunt and uncle played a crucial role by inviting Michael and his sister to live with them for a period of time while their parents worked things out. They were near enough so that there was not a continuous separation, but Michael and his sister were able to live in a non-activating environment long enough to restore their sense of safety. Michael had to make reparations for his arson and he did so appropriately, with guidance. The whole family participated in meetings that allowed Michael's behavior to be seen, over time, in the context of his military, PTSD infected family dynamics.

While Michael and his sister lived with their aunt and uncle, their parents attended workshops, and went to regular therapy individually and together. They attended a retreat that was specifically for combat survivors and their partners. They participated in a wilderness program that allowed them to be with other couples in the outdoors, where there was enough space for the complex issues of transition to be released, at least in part. Thankfully they were able to resolve the accumulation of unaddressed feelings that had built to the breaking point in their lives. Every military family should receive this quality of support.

This chapter zeroes in on the ways that we can shield children from the contaminants of war. Towards the end I comment on the marital and relational impacts of war and military life. Service children are likely one of the most neglected populations worldwide. The tragic implications of this error are evident in the statistics on traumatic repetition.[3] When we do not advocate for children, we betray ourselves and we steal their dreams. We destroy the future.

Almost half a million military children today in the United States have been diagnosed with clinical depression, and the rates of autism and learning challenges for children and youth is significantly higher in military families than in the general population worldwide.[4] According to the United States Office of Veterans Affairs, the children of veterans are exhibiting rising rates of school, family and peer related emotional and social difficulties that far outdistance the statistics for their age levels in the national sample.[5]

The family centered transition approach that Cynde Collins-Clark and I recommend in our REST House model, and the advocacy network that Joy O'Neill has built in her Service Children Support Network, would make life changing differences in the lives of military families worldwide if they were implemented. Our ideas are so obvious that when people hear about them they consistently ask, "You mean we don't already have that?"

Echoes of Silence: Why We Cannot Be Passive in the Face of Emotional Numbing

Wherever I go in the world to speak to the offspring of those who served in war, I hear this reiterated: "We never talk about it." Silence is used as a protective shield when it is actually a weapon. Given silence, children will generate their own developmentally driven assumptions that are rarely positive and usually self-demeaning. Children will inevitably take responsibility for their parents silence, rage, grief and violence. They will assume they are the cause. Their resultant compensations manipulate and drive their learning and development. The fallout may be psychological or health related, or both and it will be epigenetically transmitted to future generations if no one intervenes.

There are long-term implications to repeated exposure to

emotional numbing that I, and many other children of war, have experienced. A child cannot grasp why emotional numbing happens. Dr. Ed Tronick's "Still Face" research, first presented in 1975, clearly reveals the profound developmental consequences when a trusted caregiver is unresponsive. In his landmark studies using videotaped exchanges between children and adults, Dr. Tronick highlights how human development flourishes in an interactive, co-participatory, synchronous relational environment. On the other hand, when a child's outreach is met with stony silence, lack of response, preoccupation, distractedness, judgement or rejection, the outcomes for the child are increasing levels of stress and anxiety. The longer an adult remains unresponsive, the greater the child's distress.[6]

We already have sufficient evidence of the developmental and neurological consequences of emotional numbing for children, and these can be extended, with appropriate adaptations, to adolescents and adults. Since it has already been clearly documented that emotional numbing is a characteristic of how war comes home, the next step is to identify what we do about it to protect children, marriages and families.[7]

I was haunted for far too long by the image of my father's moody countenance that was frequently the precursor to his violent eruptions. No one intervened to tell me that my father's unresponsiveness, as well as his volatility, was unrelated to me. This deepened the mystery. Eventually the mystery became a scar on my nervous system. Fortunately I learned how to repair that scar but it took me a long time to find out how to do that. I am motivated to share the resources I discovered so that others will not respond passively to emotional numbing. The sooner the imprinting cycle of emotional numbing is interrupted the less disfiguring the scar. Indeed I believe it is entirely possible to intervene soon enough so that there is no scar at all. That is why I have written this book. When caregivers and family members are alerted to protect a child or an adolescent or even a young adult from exposures to emotional numbing, and when they have skills to reorganize the way a young person's nervous system responds, then further damages are prevented.

Adults tend to be shocked when a once personable partner, family member or friend becomes emotionally numb and remains unresponsive and altered in this way for an extended time. Adults observing this tend to be intimidated and fearful, and therefore they withdraw from the situation. They ignore it and hope it will go away. They assuage their confusion and sense of impotency by attributing the behavior to PTSD or "a phase", and they avoid the way the emotional numbing is contaminating others, freezing the expression and vitality in a home or in a family, and hurting children.

This is what comes back to me after all my years of healing and recovery. I am still left with a sense of incredulity that there was not a single individual, nor an agency, able to see what my brother and I needed when war came home to us. My mother's isolation, shame and disempowering choices increased our vulnerability. In the absence of knowledgeable, wise support, we became casualties of war, but our numbers were never counted. Today we have the capacity to change this pattern. The cumulative evidence about the repercussions of emotional numbing, combined with the validating discoveries of neuroscience, allows us to finally read the handwriting on the wall and to do something with it.

I suggest that change must come in a bottom up way, initiated by the families of veterans. We are the most immersed in what war brings home. Education. advocacy and collective action are the recipe. More and more partners of soldiers and parents of service children are speaking out about the ramifications of emotional numbing. We are building momentum for a transformation in awareness.

Three Wars/Three Families: Early Intervention

"The stress of war affects children even prior to their birth."
☐ National Center for Children in Poverty[8]

We, the families of veterans, are research scientists. Our personal and collective lives can give us the data we need to make a difference for our children. We can be the experts if we choose to investigate and pay attention. I have educated myself, for instance, by reflecting on my experience growing up as the child of a soldier with an undiagnosed Traumatic Brain Injury (TBI) and severe

Post Traumatic Stress Disorder. (PTSD). My father was missing in action when I was born as a sickly infant to a highly stressed mother. There was no preparation or family structure to support her or to nurture my physical and psychological development. My mother immediately entered a prolonged and serious postpartum depression. This was actually an extension of the depression she experienced during her pregnancy with me due to my father's deployment, his MIA status, the instability of their relationship, and her financial hardships. Research confirms that postpartum depression is more likely for mothers with deployed husbands than for mothers in the general population.[9] Knowing this, we can and should assure that pregnant wives of deployed soldiers have caregivers to support them throughout their pregnancies and during the early and critical post-natal period.

My grandfather was not an educated man but he had loving instincts and a willingness to help his daughter and new grand-daughter. He rose to the challenge out of the goodness of his heart and filled the gap in my life and my mother's life. His presence helped bring stability when otherwise there was none. Research shows that children who have a stable familial infrastructure and at least one adult who can be there for them will suffer less damage from secondary traumatization.[10] Low family cohesion increases the risk to children. The timing of when the child experiences threat and the continuity of the support available determines the magnitude of that child's stress. The internal state of the child shifts with the level and duration of threat. If a family member or someone in the community functions as an advocate, the consequences of traumatic exposures are mitigated along with the likelihood of traumatic repetition. To this day my memories of my grandfather mitigate the difficulties of my early life.

Military Children: Neurodeiversity and Community Support

When Eileen McKinley's twins were diagnosed with developmental delays her Army husband was in Vietnam. She had an older neurotypical child and now two little ones with special needs. My book, *New Frontiers in Sensory Integration,* guides

41

families through the grueling process of diagnosis, identifying therapies and adjusting to raising a neurodiverse child.[11] This is a life changing task for a two parent family with one special needs child, much less for someone who is virtually a single military parent with two children who require special services and whose husband is living in harm's way. The demands that Eileen faced almost every day were close to impossible to meet.

Eileen herself was the daughter of a military family, but that, she said, undermined rather than prepared her to have the stamina for this. Her family carried residual scars as a result of her father's service in two wars that had left him unpredictable, violent and addicted to gambling. "I hated being a military child," Eileen said. "It took away my voice and my confidence." Now facing life as a military mom she desperately wanted to protect her children from paying the price for her husband's military service. What she lacked in confidence she made up for in courage. She found her voice for her children and it changed everything. Eileen's experience reveals how military families, faced with insurmountable difficulty, find the will to blast through bureaucracy, rejection, isolation, and an appalling lack of services to do what needs to be done for their children.

Eileen knew she needed help. She could not do this alone. Even with her complaints about military life, Eileen was certain that the loyalty that military families felt for their community was reliable. Their sense of camaraderie and interconnectedness mixed with an insistence that they are indestructible make military families feisty. Eileen needed some of that spirit. She decided to allow herself to be vulnerable and reach out to others including military wives and mothers for respite.

Eileen's situation was complicated by the fact that she had delivered her children in a military hospital where the procedures were questionable, and she suspected that had contributed to the neurological issues of her twins. She had to do the research and ask the hard questions that would clarify this for her. In order to do this Eileen needed people she could trust to watch her children. She got much more than that. Her helpers cooked her meals, cleaned her house and helped her organize her notes.

While her husband grew more defeated fighting a questionable war under great social pressure, Eileen battled the institution that drafted him and gained her strength. As she fought for her children's right to have the support services they required, she found her passion. The meek, passive collapse that had shaped her response to her father's undiagnosed PTSD evaporated. Despite the odds, Eileen found herself energized rather than depleted by her circumstances.

She would need that passion because when her husband came back, he retreated into a shamed depression that cast a shadow over her home. This, however, did not stop Eileen's advocacy for her children. Now, almost forty years later, Eileen feels that fighting for her children also gave her the capacity to save her marriage. "I learned to educate myself and to not collapse because I thought I was inadequate. I had to find a way to learn about PTSD before anyone even knew what it was. My husband was a different person and I had to find out why. We had to care enough to find our way back to each other."

"My children taught me to investigate and find my own answers," Eileen continues, "and the military and civilian mothers who supported me taught me to never give up. These lessons sustained me when my husband came home and brought his war experiences with him. Having fought for my children, I knew I could fight for my marriage and my family even though the odds were against me. Today I am so glad that I made that choice."[12]

What Eileen discovered creates a model for military mothers today, encouraging them to form support groups and build their collective spirit so that no one is isolated or abandoned in their community. When Eileen asked the women around her to help there was not a single refusal. Everyone answered yes before she even completed her request. Families are a powerful force for change. Let's rally together!

Collective action and community support are viable alternatives to struggling with bureaucratic delays and agency entanglements. In places like Uganda, India and Afghanistan, a "take it to the people" model of therapy is emerging. When individuals in a village or neighborhood are educated to become lay counselors under the auspices of the World Health Organization, they have been shown to be a strong force in relieving depression and improving home and work life for people devastated by war and violence.[13] Around the world we are finding ways to care for each other out of necessity and out of the rubble of war, conflict and disaster. Community and family based mental health may well be the new frontier. I believe in that direction.

Listening to The Cry For Help

The day in April when her husband came back from Iraq was the worst day in Camille's life. John was a completely changed man who could not face what had happened to him. While Camille reeled from shock and her husband grew increasingly more isolated and withdrawn, her children slipped into destructive compensations due to their experience of family disintegration.

It would take five years to get a diagnosis of Traumatic Brain Injury (TBI) and PTSD so that John could receive services and the family could have counseling. In those five years the children entered a chaotic adolescence, John lost all capacity to earn a living, and the family home was in foreclosure. On the brink of complete collapse Camille woke up to the fact that she was living with combat shock and she either had to face it and become educated about it, or leave. She chose to stay.

Because Camille found an understanding of TBI and PTSD, and because she used this understanding to overcome her despair, she can celebrate her family today. What made the difference? Camille says she decided to really listen to the cry for help that she heard in her husband's struggle and in her children's behaviors. She realized that she had to be the one who came out of shock first. Her children needed her. Her husband needed her.

Camille stopped reacting and learned how to become an observer who reflects on what she witnesses. She had to dig deep inside herself to find the stamina and courage to change. She went on a quest to comprehend polytraumas. She innovated strategies for communication and life management. She ferreted out relational designs to meet who her husband had become. He now credits her for saving their family. Camille knows that what she did was extremely difficult; even verging on the impossible. She understands with great compassion why some families are destroyed by this process. And she knows that the healing is never over. She is still on the journey.[14]

World War II, the war in Vietnam and the war in Iraq: Three wars and still families have to pull themselves up by their bootstraps. Let the messages from these families reach into the hearts and minds of people everywhere so that the damages of war are lessened and the traumatic repetition that comes from unhealed war trauma ceases. It has fallen into our hands to do this.

Why We Must Speak Up in The Name of Our Children

Some of the greatest damages of war are epigenetic. The children of veterans are the most vulnerable to this rapidly spreading heritable infection. The contagion is erupting like a wild fire across the world. There are already a multitude of studies to demonstrate that the children of traumatized veterans exhibit a spectrum of health and developmental difficulties. In virtually all cases, when a veteran returns, a crisis ensues in that veteran's home.[15] These difficulties produce social burdens that are costly as trauma is re-enacted.

Creative strategies that families and communities implement independently are more likely to succeed than waiting for larger external agencies to act on our behalf. Thinking outside the box, identifying worthwhile alternatives, and conducting support and focus groups to problem solve as a community of people meeting the same challenges, will go a long way towards instilling positive change. Trauma increases with helplessness. Intelligent action differentiates the past from the present and empowers individuals to make a difference for themselves and for each other.

I often feel overwhelmed by the enormity of the issues facing the families of veterans, and heart-broken by what is happening to our children. But I am choosing to voice our potential and our collective resilience rather than collapsing. Whatever competence or skill I feel I lack is less important than my willingness to act. Please join me in knowing that whatever you can offer is needed. Do not hold back. We must and we will turn the tide on this century's old issue that is ready now to come to light. Consult the resource directory in Chapter Nine to link with existing networks already established for this purpose, and for encouragement in creating your own.

The Spotlight is on the Partners of Veterans

There is no question that the partners of veterans have to prepare themselves to be the ones who advocate for their children. Sometimes that is the only choice, and as Camille realized, surrendering to that can turn out to be illuminating and rewarding. The list below itemizes some of the basics needed to handle that challenge.

1. Identify support groups and attend those that are gratifying;
2. Learn and practice calming skills such as mindfulness, contemplative prayer, meditation, yoga, energy medicine or any related tools that you are comfortable with to assure stability under difficult circumstances;
3. Arrange respite for yourself in advance of needing it ;
4. Put outlets in place like exercise, music, dance and art to meet personal and expressive needs for yourself and your children;
5. Educate yourself about TBI, PTSD and related conditions as a way to Bear Witness and cultivate Resilient Empathy;
6. Learn about the brain and human development;
7. Learn about epigenetics and Secondary Traumatization and how it impacts adults and children;
8. Find ways to have fun and enjoy playful activities with your children;
9. Learn the skills that help children differentiate themselves from traumatic behavior; and
10. Above all, appreciate and love yourself for using the challenges that war brings home as routes to empowerment

Coming Home

"I know now. I know war is hard. But coming home can be harder."
☐ Amalie Flynn, *Wife and War*[16]

It is impossible in the context of this book, or perhaps in any book, to fully address the relational impacts of war. Marriages and partnerships endure enormous strain as a result of deployments and then, for those fortunate enough to return home, further strain from the stress of re-entry when everything is changed.

Because this book is oriented primarily towards families and has a special emphasis on advocating for children, the relational issues that I point to are primarily for relationships that include children. I believe that each marriage, as with each individual, needs to be understood on its own terms. Partnerships are complex, multi-faceted and intricate and they deserve personalized attention if healing is to happen.

The terrorist attacks of 9/11 and the military actions that followed them changed the tenor of many marriages. Individuals who had enrolled in the military as reservists became active duty soldiers, increasing the number of separations in families many times over around the world. We can no longer assume that soldiers sent to theaters of war are male. Mothers are deployed and leave their children in the care of their husbands, or their ex-husbands. Sometimes mothers and fathers are both deployed, and children are left with available family members. These conditions place new and previously completely unknown strains on marriages.

Virtually every service marriage that has withstood the vicissitudes of war and combat demands a healing space. Partners deserve the time and attention to rediscover who they are, and to sort out where they have been and where they have landed, both individually and as a couple. Those that come through this crucible with health merit their own medal of honor.

Central to understanding the healing journey of each marriage are degrees of wounding, both visible and invisible, and the number of deployments. Because each member of the partnership has lived such a complex, dense, multi-layered existence separately from their partner, the catch-up time will entail enormous patience and some structure. Creating a framework for reunification is in itself a mighty task given the demands of family life.

Without minimizing the enormity of the undertaking for military spouses, and out of my deep respect for it, I am called to emphasize and underscore the word compassion. Compassion for self along with compassion for the other is perhaps the only concept big enough to hold what can sustain relationships when war comes home. My parents were unprepared, in any way, to find this compassion. It did not exist for them and therefore our family was shattered. I offer the options that are in this book with the hope that I can one day say that we have come a long way since that time.

If undertaken by the non-service family member even prior to when a soldier returns, the suggestions in Chapter Seven for expressive outlets and the applied touch practices in Chapter Eight help build the patience and compassion that are needed for re-entry.Cordoning off the time and developing the discipline to maintain self-care is daunting but well worth the effort. The entire family will reap the benefits.

Service conditions have changed substantially in the post 9/11 world. Even though the War in Vietnam set the stage for our evolving definitions of PTSD, the wars in Iraq and Afghanistan turned yet another corner on the neurological, emotional, psychological and unavoidable spiritual damages of war. These inevitably transfer to intimate relationships. Nothing tests marriage vows like war. There is no part of a marriage that remains untouched by war. My prayer is that service marriages will be given the dignified support they deserve through therapeutic guidance that transcends formulas. This kind of guidance looks at the two people in the marriage, where they came from and where they are, alongside their role as sustaining cross beams in the family structure. This is what Cynde Collins-Clark and I have in mind in the REST House design.

By believing in this vision of optimum care for the families of veterans, I become a force to manifest its possibility. I do not classify this as fantasy. When people ask in reference to the REST House design, "You mean we do not already have this?" they are validating the common sense nature of what we know is needed when war comes home.

Thankfully the partners of warriors are now writing about what they have learned. I am deeply impressed by how someone like Amalie Flynn, for instance, is able to transmit the grueling internal reorganization she goes through as her marriage is shaped by war. Beginning with her direct observation of the collapse of the World Trade Center towers through to the return of her soldier husband from Afghanistan, Amalie Flynn makes known the maze-like interface between politics and intimacy, world events and the marriage bed, and how what changes melds with what endures.

Amalie and others like her are the guides that struggling partners seek in their desperation to come to grips with how war comes home. Amalie's experiences more than formulas for relational dynamics, demonstrate that we can come back to each other and simultaneously come back to ourselves. It is not easy, but it can be done.[16]

Invisible wounds are not readily detected and official diagnoses are hard to come by, even under the best of circumstances. When present, TBI, or severe PTSD which is likely due to the prevalence of polytraumas, wreak havoc on relationships and are terribly confusing. There is not a simple answer to this situation aside from advocacy for more diagnostic information and a higher quality of service. As I have reiterated throughout, self-education is a necessity, and the more empowered the individuals in a relationship are, the more accessible the remedies. Everything points to advocacy.

Chapter 3 Notes

1. Purnell, C. (2010) 'Childhood trauma and adult attachment.' *Healthcare Counseling and Psychotherapy.* April; 10:2.

2. Attachment is the emotional bond between two individuals that can form in a variety of ways. Under healthy circumstances, a child bonds with parents because there is safety and love. There are other forms of attachment, however, that occur under less healthy circumstances so that the attachment is formed through anxiety, such as when the mother's need, for instance, is met by the child rather than the reverse. Theoreticians and researchers like John Bowlby, Margaret Mahler and Ed Tronick, who I refer to in this chapter, have made essential contributions to our understanding of human development. To comprehend what happens to children in military families at various stages, beginning in utero, some education about attachment is extremely useful. This education also helps us to understand ourselves and why adults respond the way that they do to war and how it comes home.

3. University of Southern California sociologist Tamika Gilreath, commenting on her study of 2,409 students with a parent in the military that shows that 12% of the children reported suicide attempts, suicidal ideation, violent thinking or other violence such as self-harming, concludes that, "Children are bearing the burden of our wars." Her study was published in the J*ournal of European Child and Adolescent Psychiatry*, July 2015.

4. A number of independent organizations have formed to help military families living with autism. These are founded by military families who realized that the resources available to them through government agencies were insufficient and inadequate. These organizations, like Autism Care and Treatment for Military Families (also called ACT Today for Military Families) and American Military Families Autism Support Network report that the figure of 1 in 88 military children with autism is inaccurate and that the more accurate rate is 1 in 50. The contention that the numbers are increasing is difficult to substantiate for a variety of reasons including a paucity of research. Nevertheless the development of auxiliary, independent non-profits to meet the challenge of autism in military families is a new one and reflects a growing demand as well as a growing awareness of this phenomenon.

5. The Watson Institute of International and Public Affairs of Brown University in their March 2013 Costs of War report estimates that domestic violence has increased by 54% in military families and child abuse has increased by 40% since July 2010 resulting in elevated levels of stress, depression and learning challenges amongst military children in the United States.

    The Journal of the American Academy of Child and Adolescent Psychiatry reported that children show an increased risk for mental health difficulties when a military parent returns from deployment as compared to children whose parents were not deployed. Dr. Elizabeth Hisle-Gorwan of the Uniformed Services University of the Health Sciences analyzed data for 487,460 children ages 3-8. The results were published in March 2015.

6. Tronick, E. (2007) *The Neurobehavioral and Social-Emotional Development of Infants and Children.* New York: W.W.Norton & Co.

7. The link that I am suggesting between Dr. Ed Tronick's Still Face experiments and emotional numbing is unique to me. The following publications reference the defining characteristic of emotional numbing as a major contributor to Secondary Traumatization while simultaneously pointing to the paucity of research into emotional numbing. Susan L. Ray and Meredith Vanstone, Impact of PTSD and emotional numbing on veterans' family relationships, *Nursing Studies,* June 2009, Vol 46, No.6, pgs. 838-847; Todd B. Karshad et al, Anhedonia and emotional numbing in combat veterans with PTSD, *Behavioral Research and Therapy*, 2006, Vol 44, pgs. 457-467; interviews with Dr. Frank Ochberg, 2011 and 2012

8. Report on Child Development (2012). National Centre for Children in Poverty at Columbia University.

9. Interview with psychotherapist Lesley Carter who serves military families in Edinburgh, Scotland, May 2015; Jacqueline Rychnnowsky, NC USN, Screening for postpartum depression in military women with the Postpartum Depression Screening Scale, *Military Medicine,* Vol.171, Nov. 2006.

10. Resources are proliferating to assist engaged parents in preventing trauma's debilitating impacts on chilldren. I recommend Dr. Bruce Perry's Child Trauma Academy based in Houston, Texas. Dr. Perry has authored numerous books (such as *The Boy Who Was Raised As A Dog and Born for Love*) and articles that explain the neurobiology of parental presence and how it sustains a child despite traumatic exposures. He concurs with the quote that introduces this chapter that trauma does not inevitably lead to difficulty and tragedy for children. What is clear, however, is that parents have to participate in learning. In addition to Dr. Perry, my colleague Dr. Peter Levine provides a route to prepare parents to calm their own minds in order to be present for a child in his book *Trauma Through A Child's Eyes* (pgs. 71-36).

11. Mines, S. (2014) *New Frontiers in Sensory Integration: Limbic Stimulation, Authentic Relationship and a Multi-Disciplinary Treatment Design.* Stillwater, OK: New Forums Press.

12. The quotations here are derived from a personal interview conducted by the author with a military spouse and mother who prefers to remain anonymous, so a pseudonym has been used. May/June 2015.

13. Bower, B. (2013) Heal Thy Neighbor: Mental health services recruit locals to help residents of poor and war-torn countries. *Science News, 184*: 22 – 26.

14. The quotations here are derived from a personal interview and correspondence with a military spouse and mother who prefers to remain anonymous, so a pseudonym has been used. May/June 2015.

15. H.T. De Burgh et al, The impact of deployment to Iraq and Afghanistan on families of military personnel, *International Review of Psychiatry,* April 2011, Vol. 23, pgs. 192-200; *Trauma Faced by Children of Military Families*, report of the National Center of Children in Poverty of Columbia University, May 2010, by F. Sogomonyan and J.L. Cooper; G. L. Nicholson et al., Chronic mycoplasmal infection and autism in veterans' children, *Medical Veritas*, 2005, pgs. 383-387.

16. Flynn, A. (2013) *Wife and War: The Memoir.* Rhode Island, USA. www.wifeandwar.wordpress.com.

Chapter Four

Neurodiversity and the Children of War

Justin and his mother Lynn arrived thirty minutes late for their appointment with me. I had seen a long list of candidates for the clinical trials I was conducting for an autism study and they were the last family I would see that day. The clinic was near an army base and a majority of the applicants were from military families. To be considered for the study the children were required to be between the ages of four and nine years and have documentation of an autism diagnosis from their pediatrician. Only those in the mild range on the spectrum were considered. They also had to be receiving Occupational and Physical Therapy in order to qualify. Justin, who was seven years old, had passed these entry requirements and we were now at the stage of reviewing permissions and procedures.

Lynn was harried and still wearing her uniform from her job as a technical assistant in a dentist's office. Justin's younger brother Sam was in tow since mom had no choice but to bring him along. Just as we got settled Lynn's phone rang and she signaled to me that she had to leave the room. Justin and Sam, who was four, looked tired and hungry. I got out the snacks and games and they perked up, though Justin kept glancing at the door behind which his mother had disappeared. We were intent on a game of connect- the- dots when Lynn returned with a troubled look on her face, let out a sharp sigh, and sat down. The eyes of both boys darted to her immediately. Lynn ignored them, turned to me and asked, "How long is this study?"

"Two years, "I answered. "With follow up interviews at six months and a year post-study."

"Well, we will be moving before that," she retorted curtly, "So there's no point."

Startled by her pronouncement the boys and I looked at Lynn inquiringly, but she said nothing more and stared off into the distance. After a pause punctured by numerous sighs, Lynn poured out a story of overwork and relentless frustration, finally giving in to the feelings of grief and anger that were hidden behind her stoic armor.

Justin's family had moved almost every two years since he was born. He was learning about his next move while sitting in the office of someone he had just met while his mother collapsed in tears. His little brother looked like he would start crying soon too. Justin took the Legos I had brought out and began assembling them into rows. Sam was distracted by this and tried to engage with his brother but Justin pushed him away. Then Sam let out a scream and pointed at Justin. Lynn glared at them both. She made a move to smack Justin but then glanced at me and sighed yet again. "We just don't know what to do with him," Lynn said. "He won't share with his brother." Justin ignored his mother's comment and continued lining up the Legos. Sam glowered and wiped away his tears, still looking longingly at the Legos.

Common necessities in military families like high mobility ripen children for vulnerability to psychological, sensory, learning and behavioral challenges. Nevertheless a quest for research studies into how military children respond to these conditions reaps very little. In fact, there are hardly any clinical publications that focus on the neurological needs of military children and even less about what we can do to support them. Evidence does accumulate that learning and behavioral difficulties are steadily on the rise for military families worldwide, but the magnitude of the problem does not generate equally strong solution oriented proposals.[1]

Justin had been placed on the spectrum when he was five by a physician he no longer saw since his family was relocated after the diagnosis. Since then his father had deployed twice. The Physical and Occupational Therapy Justin received was through the schools he attended, all of which thankfully offered these services, but the therapists were not consistent. While his records followed him wherever he was transferred, no one was considering whether there was a relationship between his experience and his father's deployments.

Our military children are hearty souls, trying to grow and learn and make friends while everything swirls around them. They walk the very thin line between trauma and neurodiversity, navigating at every step the emotional intensity in their homes. Their stories are largely untold. Nevertheless these children and youth are heroic. They are subjected to enormous pressures during their crucial developmental years. They live in a world of shifting locations and circumstances and they can be in the direct line of fire when war comes home. Their needs are not highlighted in agency services even though they are the most vulnerable to the circumstances of war and have the fewest resources. Despite an underlying assumption that wars are somehow fought for children, they pay an incalculable price for them.

What can parents do to protect their children from psychological damage and sensory and learning difficulties? Often the non-service parent, like Justin's mother, is so overcome by responsibility that he or she cannot slow down enough to focus on the children. My book, *New Frontiers in Sensory Integration,* is a primer for parents on how to optimize the potential of children with sensory needs like Justin's.[2] It defines what sensory needs are and how these can evolve out of a mix of trauma and neurological development. Children are always doing their best to succeed and function even when their nervous systems are overwhelmed and sensory deficits impair them. A child who is struggling with reading, for instance, may have a visual processing difficulty that is the product of stress at home. Sorting out these variables is an intricate task and parents have to steer it on the basis of their knowledge of their child. Diagnostic labels can be Band-Aids on more complex, and sometimes much simpler, conditions. Most people are encultured to accept diagnostics too readily and in so doing they lose sight of the child.

Military families can use the chapters of *New Frontiers in*

Sensory Integration as life rafts to learn how they can anchor their children through the way that they interact with them, and reel them in from reactions to the permutations of military life. Justin was able to play with his brother, for example, when the situation was structured and focused, providing the containment that he needed. Consistent non-punitive boundary enforcement always enhances potential. Justin was intelligent, sensitive, receptive and completely tuned in to the emotional dynamics around him.

As I listened to Lynn, Justin and Sam that day I could hear their plea for help. Another move without a change in awareness for this family could seal in dysfunctional compensatory behaviors that were clearly at play. Justin was a remarkable boy who was being labeled as the problem when in fact he was absorbing the difficulties that were circulating around him. I had something useful to offer this family and I felt obligated to share it. After all, there had to be a reason why they were here with me at the end of the day when I had time to be of service to them.

New Frontiers in Sensory Integration encourages parents to investigate how their words and actions are building their children's brains. If parents allow themselves to separate from other pressures and be fully present to their children, it is amazing how much easier it is to manage behavior and find connection. Simple presence stabilizes children. Parents are always surprised to see how much better it feels to attune to their children rather than criticize them. Attunement lessens the necessity for control. A distracted environment, as Justin's had been for some time, contributed to his feeing of disconnection.

Sensory disturbances result when the primary sensory systems cannot mediate or filter input from the external world. If, for instance, a child is overwhelmed by shifting conditions in their environment, they may react by becoming defensive, or by shutting down to touch or other sensory experience. This shutting down can be diagnosed as autism, which is a form of neurodiversity or neurological difference, but it likely has a sensory component. The child is using his senses to compensate for something uncontrollably painful. From this example you can see how difficult it is to distinguish psychological, sensory and neurodevelopmental issues. Add to this conundrum the complex dynamics of military life and war and you can see the necessity for careful, calm and focused attention for each child.

Just as polytraumas are neurologically debilitating for soldiers, so too are they for children. Sensory issues may arise as coping mechanisms, and then be exacerbated by high mobility and repeated deployments coupled with loss of family and friends, putting the child at risk. In the maze of the military lifestyle this accumulation of traumas can go undetected. The longer these issues are left to smolder, the more severe they become. It is because of this that I endeavor to educate parents about sensory needs, early intervention and home based strategies. Even when a family's location changes, the parent's attunement and attention can be the constant that creates nervous system stability.

Joy O'Neill's model of the Service Children Support Network goes a step further. She has developed a structure for unifying the family and the school system in the context of military culture. Her recommendation for a tracking system for each child makes all the sense in the world. Without an anchor, children drift, seeking something with which to bond. This is one of the seeds of addictions.

As an educator as well as a military spouse and mother Joy O'Neill is thoroughly qualified to comment on the learning impacts of high mobility, deployment and other components of a child's experience in a military family. Her Service Children Support Network (SCSN) that is currently functioning in her local community in Buckinghamshire, England, addresses the need of service children to have a consistent, knowledgeable advocate who knits together their home and educational experiences. The interruptions in attachment that mark military life are not only balanced by Joy's paradigm, they also lessen the burden for military parents.

This model can be translated anywhere in the world. Through a Family Support Coordinator who facilitates communication between schools, families and community agencies, a child is held and guided throughout their learning experience. Fragmentation is averted. Joy's pilot studies show how effective and well received these concepts are.[3]

High mobility and high stress scramble a young person's learning so that their ability to focus and sustain basic academic skills like reading or healthy social engagement suffers. It becomes difficult under these circumstances to differentiate learning challenges from sensory issues; neurological issues from emotional and psychological needs. In the hailstorm of demands that can intermittently shape a military household, it may be confusing to ascertain if the child is reacting to the difficulties of mobility or deployments, or if they are caught in the crosshairs of different school systems, or all of the above. Someone needs to be in charge of making these inquiries with a singular focus on the child and usually the non-service parent is too distracted to do this, especially if there are other children in the household.

How To Determine if a Child is a Candidate for Sensory Evaluation

The characteristics that Justin exhibited and that resulted in his autism diagnosis would also suggest a need for a sensory evaluation. Parents need to be sensitive to these traits and how to address them. These include:

1. Withdrawing from interaction with other children at school. Justin even backed out of play with his same age cousins when they got together;
2. Preferring solitary play and sometimes obsessively lining up toys;
3. Though Justin's hearing had been tested as normal, he did not respond to instructions;
4. Justin did not express his feelings directly;
5. Justin was more serious than playful;
6. Justin was not interested in a variety of toys or activities but seemed to prefer to repeat the same ones; and
7. He was not reading or speaking on a par with his peers.

Justin's mother and father knew that something was not right but they tended to attribute that more to Justin's resistance. They were not aware of when Justin did engage in healthy play, or what was happening for him when he did not.

Justin's parents were frustrated by the relocations and the complications of uprooting the children from their activities over and over again, but they saw this as part and parcel of the military lifestyle in which they were both raised. They were not aware of the developmental implications for their children of these disruptions. Explaining these things to them in a way they could comprehend was a high priority. Indeed it was the game changer for Justin, Sam and their family. What follows summarizes what I shared with them.

The Art and Joy of Limbic Stimulation

As I discuss in my book, *New Frontiers in Sensory Integration*, the limbic brain mediates between the survival and executive brains.[4] The limbic brain grows healthy in response to engaged stimulation and the loving attuned presence of the adults in the child's world. When the limbic brain is vital and resilient, making good decisions is natural. Justin was not making good decisions in his exchanges with others, including his teachers and peers. This interrupted and delayed his learning. He was unable to connect in ways that were expected of him, like sharing with his brother. I suggested the possibility that this mirrored the ways in which he did not feel connected. Perhaps the physical absence of his father and the consequent pressures that distracted his mother were playing a part in Justin's difficulties. There were two simple things that I suggested Justin's parents do to tease his limbic brain into novel tracks:

1. Discover what really interested and enthralled their son; and
2. Engage in that activity with him.

What Justin really liked was building things. He liked to find out how things worked. He was quietly curious rather than bombarding his parents with questions. When he wanted to explore the mechanics of something, like a fan for instance, he watched it for a long time. I suggested to Justin's father that he notice when Justin was watching something and then without saying anything, begin to take it apart while Justin was watching. This worked! Justin and his dad first silently assembled a clock, and then a radio, and by the time they got to the vacuum cleaner, they were talking to each other about how to do it.

 Seeing life through Justin's eyes eventually stirred a change of heart for his parents. It was as if they were seeing him afresh. Underneath his aggression and withdrawal they saw that he was someone precious and vulnerable who was in pain because his legitimate need for both a mother and a father to guide and protect him was frustrated. When Justin's parents stopped defending the necessity for Justin to adhere to their plans, a position that had consistently failed, new options occurred to them that they had never considered before.

Justin's father discovered that the military has an obligation to assign families to areas where appropriate services for their children are available, and to allow them to remain in those areas for a minimum of five years.[5] If children have special needs, high mobility is a great disadvantage to them. As I could see even in my first meeting with Justin, mobility exacerbated his difficulties. The news that he would be relocating aroused both his withdrawal and his negativity towards his brother, though Justin himself would not be able to identify the connection. That observation is an insight that requires more mature intelligence.

In the US there are complex steps that families have to go through to vouch for their special needs child, such as enrolling in the Exceptional Family Member Program (EFMP). Other countries likely have similar steps that must be taken to guarantee that you will not be relocated because it is detrimental to a child. The crucial information is that there are alternatives to being stuck with repeated mobility when you have a neurodiverse child who is damaged by it. While this alternative is not readily made available and must be sought out and pursued, it nevertheless exists and Justin's dad found it.

Military families are already so mired in bureaucracy they loathe taking on more. Asking for special services can have negative consequences in the military anywhere in the world, as soldiers who have sought help for PTSD or partners seeking relief from domestic violence have found. It is unfortunate that so much paperwork and so many steps are required in order to receive the mental health and learning support that families rightfully deserve to address the unique and complex challenges that are inherent in military life. A consistent and universal commitment to child advocacy, the core of this book's message, is what will turn the tide.

Home Based Help for Service Children with Special Needs

There are two primary avenues for the nervous system to travel on when it has to compensate for sensory overload. One uses the sympathetically driven path of adrenalizing that is characterized by fighting, reacting and hyperactivity. This is sometimes referred to by sensory professionals as "over-responsiveness." The other direction is parasympathetic, and instead of reacting, it relies on withdrawing, collapsing, becoming isolated or lethargic, and hiding. This can be called "under-responsiveness." The parasympathetic avenue usually drowns out adrenaline with cortisol, so that there is a flattening of affect and a slowing down of responses. Both dominances take a toll on health by repeatedly using neurohormones when they are no longer necessary for survival. Interestingly, veterans are caught in at this same forked road when they return home.

Justin, for instance, used the parasympathetic arm of his nervous system predominantly. I discuss this simple but revelatory paradigm of sympathetic and parasympathetic dominance for adults in my book, *We Are All in Shock*, and for children in *New Frontiers in Sensory Integration*.[6]

By learning to identify whether a child is sympathetic dominant (over-responsive) or parasympathetic dominant (under-responsive), parents and other family members can easily support a child's nervous system to find balance. They can do this at home using applied touch as well as attuned language in their interactions. For instance, you can calm a tendency to be hyperactive by placing the palms of the hands on the calves of the child's legs. Alternately, you can place your hands on the tops of their shoulders This application is also illustrated in Chapter Eight as a soothing intervention for over-stimulation. This is called Site #11 in the applied touch system described in Chapter Eight. It is used to take off burdens of over-responsibility that may be the source of the child's hyperactivity.

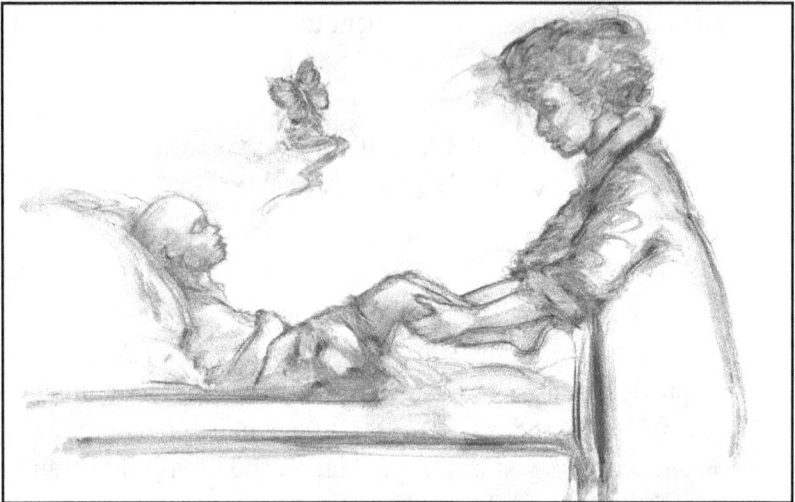

Figure 4.1a – Palming the Calves

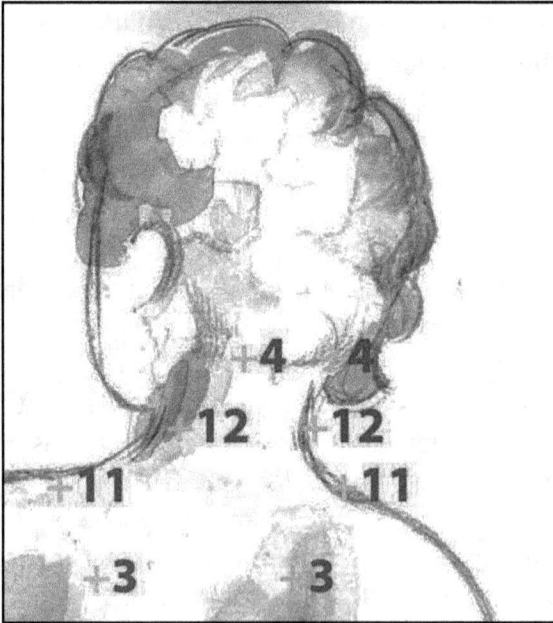

Figure 4.1b – Site #11

You can bring a child out of a withdrawn state by placing the palms of the hands on their lower back (Site #23), over the area where the kidneys are. This relieves the fatigue the child may be experiencing. These are basic supports. See Chapter Eight for additional information about how sites on the body can be held to help you and your family when war comes home.

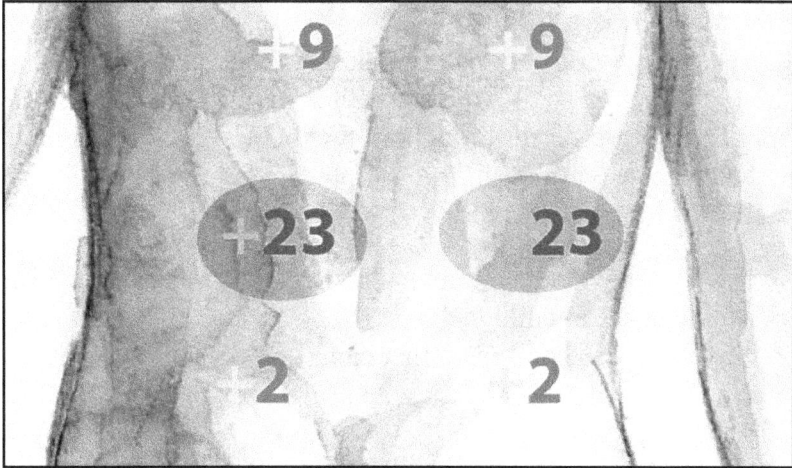

Figure 4.2 – Site #23

While we wait for family centered transition facilities like the REST House to emerge, we can rally as an international community to protect, recognize and celebrate our heroic service children and their families. Their inclusion in our awareness is a point of entry for their healing. Service families generally feel left out, and they are. The growing literature by service family members that often includes experiences with their children is making a difference. In my interviews with the parents of service children, they shared uniquely creative interventions they have developed to help their children deal with anger, grief, loss and anxiety. I would like to collect these innovative strategies to deliver them to other service families. Our successes build the most practical and effective skill bank for what children need when war comes home.

Who are The Children of War?

The goal of this chapter is to lessen developmental damages and enhance learning and growth for children while simultaneously mitigating traumatic repetition. The term "children of war" applies both to service children and children who are living in the midst of war, including refugees, immigrants, and children orphaned by war. These children are all extremely vulnerable to virtually inevitable sensory and learning difficulties that interfere significantly in their ability to grow, develop and live healthy, productive lives.

The suggestions and interventions in this book will benefit these children as well as those with a military affiliation. The applications presented throughout this book can be adjusted in virtually any environment. Two simple things are required for the delivery of these resources:

1. The presence of one or more adults who can be fully attentive to the needs of children; and
2. A relatively peaceful space that includes a comfortable place to sit with a child or children with the least distraction possible.

I have delivered applied touch resembling what is portrayed in this book along with dialogue tailored for children such as story-telling on buses, in fields, on playgrounds, in tents, in the midst of other activities, while seated with them on the ground and in makeshift homes. A perfect clinical environment or a separate room is not always available or necessary.

Serving children who have suffered the extremes of war can require additional levels of learning and training, though there is much to be said for a warm hearted presence, attuned listening and respect for the intelligence and sensitivity of the child. Dr. Bruce Perry who created the Child Trauma Academy provides education that I respect for those interested in developing more skill.[7]

Humanity must step up as the larger family for all the children of war. We are their stewards and they deserve that we be trusted mentors for them. The story of Justin in this chapter is intended to serve as a model for a child from a military family since this is the focus of this book. I do wish to offer, however, the possibility of translating his predicament and the applications in this book for a larger community of the children of war.

Justin's situation depicts how a child's true needs can become obscured in the weaving of military life with learning. Neurodiversity is a reflection of the brain's resiliency in adapting to developmental challenges. When adults take responsibility for discovering how trauma can interfere with growth, a sizable burden is taken off the shoulders of children.

Chapter 4 Notes

1. Chandra, A., et al. (2010) 'Children on the Homefront: The experience of Children from Military Families.' *Pediatrics* Jan, 125:16-25; Gregory, G., MD. (2010) 'Wartime Military Deployment and Increased Pediatric Mental and Behavioral Health Complaints.' *Pediatrics* Nov, 126(6) 1058-1066; Richardson, A., et al. (2011) 'Effects of Soldiers' Deployments on Children's Academic Performance and Behavioral Health.' RAND Center for Military Health and Policy; Yazbak, R.E., MD. (2008) Report to the National Health Federation on Autism Rates among Military Children, July 9.

2. Mines, S. (2014) *New Frontiers in Sensory Integration: Limbic Stimulation, Authentic Relationship and a Multi-Disciplinary Treatment Design.* Stillwater, OK: New Forums Press.

3. O'Neill, J. (2011) *Service Children: A Guide for Education and Welfare Professionals.* Bedfordshire, England. Authors on Line.

4. Mines, S. (2014) *New Frontiers in Sensory Integration: Limbic Stimulation, Authentic Relationship and a Multi-Disciplinary Treatment Design,* Chapter 3; pgs 43 – 57. Stillwater, OK: New Forums Press.

5. In the US this is the 2010 National Defense Authorization Act/Office of Community Support for Military Families with Special Needs. Similar acts exist in other countries for families with special needs but they have to be identified, investigated and advocated for in order to be used. The military will not necessarily inform families that these options are available.

6. Mines, S. (2003) *We Are All In Shock: How Overwhelming Experiences Shatter You...And What You Can Do About It,* Chapter 2, pgs 37 – 62. NJ: The Career Press; Mines, S. (2014) *New Frontiers in Sensory Integration: Limbic Stimulation, Authentic Relationship and a Multi-Disciplinary Treatment Design,* Chapter 5, pgs 85 – 94. Stillwater, OK: New Forums Press.

7. Dr. Bruce Perry, Child Trauma Academy. CTA is a not-for-profit organization based in Houston, Texas working to improve the lives of high-risk children through direct service, research and education. The mission of the Child Trauma Academy is to help improve the lives of traumatized and maltreated children by improving the systems that educate, nurture,

protect and enrich these children. They focus their efforts on education, service delivery, program consultation, research and innovations in clinical assessment/treatment. www.childtrauma.org.

Chapter Five

Signature Wounds and Family Implications

"Emotion is a central organizaing process within the brain."
☐ Daniel Siegel[1]

TBI's and their interaction with other traumas is a no-man's land. The spectrum of possible behavioral, emotional and psychological outcomes when polytraumas are involved is endless. To further frustrate the predicament we are in regarding signature wounds, they are more often than not undiagnosed. Family members are thus put in the position of figuring it out. Once a diagnosis is received, government agencies sometimes provide help but receiving a diagnosis is easier said than done. Some families do not know how to undertake or complete that process and are not sure when or if they should initiate it. For these and many more reasons a general education about these signature wounds is essential for all military families.

The term "polytrauma" has both current and generic definitions. Broadly it means a multiplicity of traumas and in this regard in applies to families as well as to soldiers. Children, for instance, are subjected to polytraumas when a parent is deployed, they are required to relocate, the family is fragmented and their non-service parent is depressed. In relationship to the wars in Iraq and Afghanistan, however, the term "polytraumas" is used to describe multiple wounding from explosive events that usually include a head injury. In both cases, polytraumas demand a high level of integrative, sensitive and individuated care. For soldiers, this is provided once the diagnosis is certain. For families, this is rarely provided.

In writing this book I have been compelled to revisit the way that undiagnosed polytraumas wreaked havoc in my home and stole my father from me along with my childhood. Nothing brings that more to the forefront than looking at how undiagnosed head injuries spiral out of control and spread chaos. The fallout that is most destructive lands on the developmental paths of children. This has always been true.

Sixty years separate my childhood from Shelby Garcia's. Her father returned from the War in Iraq and mine returned from World War II with undiagnosed head injuries and severe PTSD. Our families were fractured. Our little brothers were alienated and lost. Our mothers were shocked into disbelief and panic. Only through our valiant self-initiated efforts could we reconstruct ourselves. In Shelby's case a local Vet Center, one of the few informal off-base clinics for US veterans that invites families to participate, made the difference. Retroactively and with great perseverance I was able finally to uncover the mystery of what happened in my home. Shelby and I dug ourselves out of the quagmire of polytraumas.

For Shelby and I, understanding and healing came long after massive damage had already occurred. Our early development was thwarted. Our families reeled from the violence in our homes. The daily madness was unnerving. No one was unscathed. Much of this was preventable. Shelby and I are at work today to put a stop to these unnecessary losses.

In 1985 I found myself in the position of being an advocate for people with head injuries in my doctoral internship at an independent living center. Here I learned what life is like from the standpoint of a person with invisible wounds living in a culture blind to their condition. Often I was required to present my client's point of view when one of them lashed out so violently that they were arrested. In a way that I never could have predicted, I was indoctrinated into empathy and compassion for my father. Seeing through the eyes of people with neurological disabilities allowed me to forgive my father. My doctoral program thus became a spiritual cleansing and a psychological transformation.

My clients taught me how it feels to live with invisible wounds amongst people who do not want to see you at all. The internal tensions that build when there is no relief, remedy or support can be likened to stoking a volcano, preparing it every moment to erupt. As a curious and resourceful doctoral candidate I was motivated to find solutions for people who resembled my father, at least in their behavior. This was a remarkably bittersweet period marked by astounding productivity. I was piecing together an understanding of TBI and correlating that with my observations of my father to put together the pieces of the puzzle of what war brings home to families in general, and what it brought home to my family in particular.

The therapies that I developed as an outcome of this internship shaped the theoretical basis of my doctoral dissertation.[2] In 2010 these interventions were clinically tested by a group of my students at the University of Colorado.[3] While these therapies do not cure Traumatic Brain Injury, they do, as the research shows, lower stress levels, improve quality of life, memory and attention, and cultivate an increased relaxation response. The interventions tested in the 2010 study resemble those provided in Chapter Eight of this book. They can be administered at home and translate easily into self-care. They can make life better for people living with TBI and their families. Even if you only suspect that TBI might be an issue, there is no harm in using these interventions. They have no negative side effects. They can only be beneficial. They do require patience and the discipline to use them regularly as the benefits are cumulative. These include clearer thought processes, enhanced learning and understanding, and increased focus and calm.

What is striking about my doctoral research and the clinical trials from the University of Colorado is that the applications are simple, can be used by anyone, and have exceptional outcomes. Their success demonstrates that family members have within their hands the capacity to make a real difference in health outcomes. We do not have to be victimized by poor or non-existent diagnostic procedures or the absence of needed and appropriate counseling in institutions mired in bureaucracy and politics. It does take diligence, curiosity, attention, and perseverance but we can harness our powers of intelligence and intention and in so doing improve physical and mental wellbeing.

Finding person-centered care for head injury is almost as difficult today as it was when I began my doctoral studies. Left to their own devices veterans with TBI crumple into a losing confrontation with their guilt, their lack of self-worth, and their weakness in judgement. The frustrated explosions like those that occurred regularly in my childhood home send children into a tailspin, leaving them ashamed and unable to ever invite playmates home. This is how I grew up but it is not what I will tolerate for future generations because I know it does not have to be that way.

My father's head injury was responsible for his random disappearances, sometimes for extended periods, as well as his verbal, physical and sexual abuses. Once I could clearly attribute his violence to his physiology, a suffocating weight of self-denigration that I had carried for most of my life was lifted. I was freed to be the gifted person I always was, capable of making a contribution to humanity.

Certain observable behaviors are indicators of a likely closed head injury. Educating partners and other family members to be aware of these indicators and providing them with support and resources for how to take care of themselves is life changing. These include:

1. Differentiating themselves from TBI driven behaviors;
2. Learning when and how to find diagnostic and counseling assistance;
3. Enumerating ways of keeping themselves and their children safe;
4. Itemizing the options for treatment of TBI;
5. Respecting the care-giving role; and
6. Providing home-based strategies that are helpful for people with TBI and polytraumas as well as for the Secondary Traumatization that is virtually inevitable for caregivers.

Culturally sensitive and individually focused education and guidance regarding signature wounds can save the hearts, minds, spirits and, in some cases, the lives of the families of veterans. Given the frequency of polytraumas education about being proactive should be mandatory. Empowering families to be informed and aware is common sense and cost-effective.

Possible Indicators of Closed Head Injury or TBI

Individuals who have a closed head injury or Traumatic Brain Injury (TBI) may demonstrate some or all of the following characteristics:

1. Difficulties with memory;
2. Difficulties with attention;
3. Slow processing of information;
4. Disconnection, dissociation and emotional detachment;
5. Visual impairment;
6. Hearing loss;
7. Heightened irritation, frustration and anxiety;
8. Inability to be intimate;
9. Fatigues easily;
10. Erratic mood swings;
11. Sudden outbursts of anger;
12. Alterations in gait and mobility;
13. Dizziness, instability in standing, lack of physical balance;
14. Poor concentration;
15. Irrationality;
16. Obsessiveness;
17. Slurred speech;
18. Stammering or stuttering;
19. Slow language processing; and
20. Withdrawal.

The Sooner, The Better

Early detection and early treatment prevents the deepening of invisible wounds and their transmission to innocent bystanders. At the minimum, families need to know that wounded warriors will likely feel shame about their deficits, and this shame, along with the absence of treatment, will drive their injuries deeper. People with head injuries are acutely sensitive and reactive, and family members deserve to know how to protect themselves and seek assistance.

Invisible wounds suggest a mask. The person appears strong; indeed they are often aggressive, but they actually feel weak. This is a set-up for addiction as a way to mask multiple layers of confusion, pain and fear. At the bottom of this layering is a desire for human connection, a longing to be relieved of the burden of pretense. Skill and compassion, indeed mastery is needed to touch into this complexity. Some of the most highly trained professionals in the world have been unable to do so. Family members need to reach deeply into their own hearts and receive mentorship from others who have walked in these shoes in order to be able to care for someone with polytraumas.

Polytraumas call for multiple modalities and highly individualized attention. Formulaic approaches have already proven themselves unsuccessful. In her heart-wrenchingly honest portrayal of how her husband was not served by these formulas, Kayla Williams exposes another path of healing; one resembling what is recommended here, for both the wounded warrior and the caregiver. Her book, *Plenty of Time When We Get Home: Love and Recovery in the Aftermath of War,* is an intimate portrait of the impacts of TBI, PTSD and polytraumas on relationships.[4]

Polymorphous Polytraumas

When polytraumas occur in current theaters of war as a result of an explosive device or blast the medical services that are provided are the most advanced available. They save lives. Polytraumas in this category are carefully identified as needing integrative, family centered care. This is recognized by the Department of Defense, the Veterans Administration and the National Council on Disability in America.[5]

The diversity of polytraumas differentiates the damages to veterans from contemporary wars from those fought earlier. Correspondingly this means that the challenges for families and caregivers are also of another order of magnitude. Polytraumas and their consequences cannot be predicted or charted. For instance, the interface between TBI caused by exposures to blasts and IEDs, combined with sexual abuse for a female soldier, results in a brand of wounding that has not been researched or sufficiently documented. In her book, *Soldier Girls*, author Helen Thorpe follows this combo, tracking it for years, showing how it plays out in the lives of her interviewees.[6]

In its oversight hearing on TBI, the Veterans Administration admitted that despite legislation to enhance services in the United States like the Veterans Traumatic Brain Injury and Health Improvements Act of 2007, "current efforts are inadequate to insure the psychological health of our veterans." Factors like "insufficient attention to prevention," "limited access to services," and "a lack of cultural competency for diverse military populations" put soldiers, and therefore their families, at risk.[7]

Another stunning admission of this report is that without the support of dedicated loved ones, veterans with polytraumas will have no choice but to be confined to nursing homes in order to get the care they need. The uncompensated attendance and advocacy of family members, such as Abe's family whose saga you read about in Chapter One, is a life saving grace.

"Polytrauma is a new phenomenon," says Lucille Beck, Director of the Veterans Administration Office of Rehabilitation Services. "Medicine has not caught up with it."[8]

Given the ubiquity of polytraumas, families deserve not only support, financial compensation and preparatory education, they also merit access to the kinds of resources contained in this book that make a difference on a daily basis and improve the quality of life for veterans, their children and their family members. Knowing that even the medical profession is baffled by the polytraumas produced by current war conditions, family members can feel more confident to look outside the box and find what works. Mentorship from those who have walked in their shoes, like Kayla Williams, might be the best possible resource.

Polytraumas and Family Relationships

"Too long a sacrifice can make a stone of the heart."
☐ William Butler Yeats

Service members who once managed complex responsibilities and hundreds of troops find themselves suddenly unable to make change or balance a checkbook. This is how polytraumas are revealed in the nitty gritty, day to day home life .that de facto becomes the ultimate diagnostic of invisible wounds. Shamed by these paradoxes wounded warriors go into hiding, self-medicate with substances, and generally enter a steep decline that ravages family relationships. This often leads to divorce. Divorce rates are higher amongst the military than in the general population and higher still amongst veterans with polytraumas, especially TBI's.[9]

The demise of a marriage can be ugly; even brutal. Children must be protected at all costs. When they witness or even overhear altercations the ramifications reverberate through generations. If other family members can provide sanctuary for children and give partners the space to sort through the complexities of how lives are changed by polytraumas, strategies may emerge.

Three things can be said with certainty regarding polytraumas:

1. They necessitate a long term recovery process;
2. They dramatically shift family dynamics; and
3. They call for commitment and creativity from partners and family members.

Some families unravel under the strain of these demands. There can be no judgment on this outcome. The burdens and lack of compensation for them produces a heavy weight. Even the most abundant hearts can be emptied by the force of over-giving.

Bob Woodruff, the television journalist wounded in Iraq and diagnosed with TBI and PTSD, noted that "everyone processes everything in a different way" when commenting on the impacts of polytraumas on his own family life. [10]

The signature of war is written everywhere. It summons us to harness creativity to pick up the puzzle pieces. Without the clarity of intention, such as what I propose in the Caregiver Steward's Creed in Chapter One, we are vulnerable to unforeseen forms of traumatic repetition. Nothing is more daunting than the ubiquity of polytraumas. It is because of this that I propose a larger body of wisdom such as the fusion of Western neuroscience with alternative therapies to meet the challenge.

Chapter 5 Notes

1. Siegel, D. (2012), *The Developing Mind: How Relationships and the Brain Interact to Shape Who We Are.* New York: Guilford Press.

2. Mines, S. (1987) 'That Feeling of Not Being Seen as a Whole: Holistic Therapy and People with Disabilities'. Dissertations International. 48:6

3. Mc Fadden,K.L., Healy, K.M., Detterman, M.L., Kaye, J.J., Ito, T.A., Hernandez, T.D. (2011) Acupressure as a Non – Pharmacological Intervention for Traumatic Brain Injury. *Journal of Neurotrauma*, Jan; 28(1):21-34

4. Williams, K. (2014) *Plenty of Time When We Get Home: Love and Recovery in the Aftermath of War.* New York: W.W Norton & Co.

5. National Council on Disability, March 4, 2009 Report on Invisible Wounds: PTSD and TBI; Department of Defense Task Force on Mental Illness, Committee on Veterans Affairs Report to the United States Senate, May 5, 2010

6. Thorpe, H. (2014) *Soldier Girls: The Battles of Three Women at Home and at War.* New York: Scribner

7. Committee on Veterans Affairs Report to US Senate, May 5th, 2010.

8. Committee on Veterans Affairs Report to US Senate, May 5th, 2010.

9. Arango-Lasprilla, J.C., Ketchum, J.M., Dezfulian, T., et al (2008) Predictors of marital stability two years following traumatic brain injury. Brain Injury 22(7-8): 565-574; Kruetzer, J.S., et al (2007) Marital stability after brain injury: an investigation and analysis. *NeuroRehabilitation 22*(1), 53-59.

10.Interview with Bob Woodruff, "Brain Injury: My Road to Recovery." CBS Television, 2013

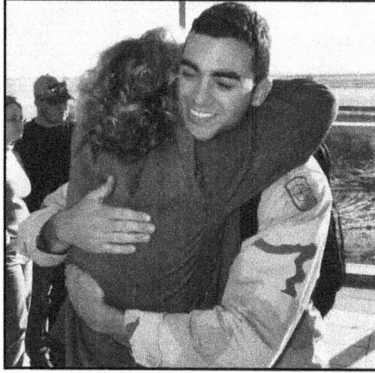

Section II
Enlightened Home Strategies

Chapter Six

The Art of Respite: Rituals of Regeneration for Caregivers

"The most challenging and important moments in healing are when we find ways to be still."
☐ Anonymous

I am devoting an entire chapter to the concept of respite because without it, long term caring for the wounds of war is close to impossible. The simplest definition of respite is that it is an interval of rest or relief. But for the partners and family members of veterans respite goes beyond that. It is the space to reclaim personal identity.

For the purposes of this book I am augmenting the definition of respite to include the discovery of personal context, direction and meaning when war has rearranged life and relationships. Respite in this light becomes the sanctuary of wholeness that counters the splintering and fragmenting forces of war. When war's unresolved suffering arrives in a civilian home it strikes a deafening chord. The scope of pain is shattering; it is like facing a veritable mountain of agony. Even those of us who experience this secondarily feel impotent to make a difference.

The moral scarring made by war's horrors makes it seem self-indulgent and even wasteful to carve out personal time. But the opposite is true. Respite is essential under these circumstances. It is the greatest hope. The practice of taking respite is what brings sustainability to caregiving and assures its longevity.

Experiencing true self-care is palpably nourishing. The first step is to identify what self-care means to you. If you have not yet found your self-care resources you may have to chart a deliberate quest to find them. Options are suggested in the chapters that follow. As you explore, know that your brand of respite will always be utterly unique to you. It is your particular medicine. Once you find it you will be fed by it for your lifetime.

Partners and caregivers for wounded warriors need regularly scheduled rituals of regeneration. If you are also a parent this statement is in boldface and underscored. Life's topographies are rearranged; relationships are scrambled; visions for the future are displaced when war comes home. We know now that soldiers are not given adequate transition resources before they re-enter family life. What most of us have thought should be automatic transition service has never existed. Facing this squarely and realistically demands that we rally intelligence and creativity. Partners and family members are the most important people in the lives of veterans in these circumstances. Our health is of the highest priority. Respite that allows us to find focus and direction is a pre-requisite to charting the path of recovery. The modes you find for your unique respite are your rituals of regeneration.

A 2007 longitudinal study of the transition of 88,000 soldiers who served in Iraq revealed that partners of veterans who understand the dynamics of their situation, and who can apply meaning to it, create real mediation at home.[1] This proactive, protective and family-affirming stance is a strong preventative to allay dysfunction. Partners can more easily find their ground if they program respite into their lives in advance; even before soldiers return home.

What Stops Us from Taking Respite?

The common characteristics of what prevents us from moving courageously in the direction of respite are:

1. Guilt;
2. Shame; and the
3. Inability to ask for help which is driven by guilt and shame.

The first step towards respite is the dissolution of guilt and shame. If you combine equal measures of guilt and shame you have the recipe for self-sabotage. Guilt is the belief that we have done something wrong and shame is the feeling that we ourselves are wrong. Guilt and shame thrive in a vague, unconscious haze that thwarts us from moving forward; we feel mysteriously flawed, unworthy and unable to clearly see ahead. We become habituated to this confusion. Caregivers get stuck in this morass because they carry not only their own historical lineages of guilt and shame; they can also unwittingly absorb layer after layer of guilt and shame from those they care for as they try dutifully to be of service.

Shedding this muggy state requires a force field; a "just do it" whoosh of motivation. Think of what you have to do to defog your car window when driving in a storm. You turn on a condenser that forces a gust of air directly at the misty surface and then you can see where you are going. Translate this into overcoming resistance and what you get is the direct action needed to ask for help by calling a friend or colleague to cover your time, watch your children, or help with tasks and research so that you can take respite. It could also mean connecting with a community agency or church organization that will assist you in identifying these helpers. As you "just do it" by reaching out, you are simultaneously shedding guilt and shame. Every caregiver deserves respite. It is the topmost item in the Caregiver Bill of Rights.

Caring for wounded warriors does resemble driving in a storm. Not having clarity is dangerous. Sometimes the best thing you can do for the safety of your family is to pull over and ask for help. Self-sabotage is a volatile state. Rage is often the most ready outlet for the layers of frustration that accumulate. Cultural conditions, including those in the military, can enforce self-sabotage. Courage is the force field that repudiates guilt and shame so that we create new conditions and stop repeating the same old defeats. It is only then that new growth is possible.

The roots of guilt and shame are deep, entangled and hardy. Vulnerabilities are often hidden in the soil of these structures. Once exposed to air and light these can be transmuted into strengths rather than hidden as weaknesses. It takes courage to test this hypothesis. Guilt and shame are frequently defenses against enormous grief and the weight of impotence when we are or were unable to stop something horrible from happening. Survivor's guilt fits this description and caregivers struggle with this as much as soldiers. Survivor's guilt feeds trauma just as sugar feeds cancer. It is a contaminant. It serves the function of self-sabotage by hampering, even forbidding, growth and change.

"Unworthy" is the word that sums up the end product of guilt and shame and unworthiness is also responsible for resistance to taking respite. It too needs to be unmasked for what it is: self-sabotage. Caregivers and family members may feel they are "less" than the soldier who endured war and combat. The feeling of unworthiness, under all circumstances, is a false belief. No one is unworthy. Though some social networks may profit from projecting unworthiness onto others, the state of unworthiness is an imposition that deserves only to be cast aside. Whatever causes us to be subservient, to squelch our own vitality or to lose identity must be rejected. Rituals of regeneration are designed for this task.

What Does Respite Look Like?

Taking respite invites us to do what appears incongruous when we are in caregiving mode. It invites us to stop. Caregivers become entrained to the rhythms of not stopping. We feel we have to keep going, no matter what. This is the well-worn path to Secondary Traumatization and its byproduct: burnout. It seems contradictory to consider respite when there is so much that remains undone. However, the truth is that the "to do list" will go on forever. There is no end to it no matter how much you do. You cannot wait until the list has nothing on it because that time will never come. Taking respite will not make the list grow longer. In fact, surprisingly, it could help shorten the list.

Stopping is rebooting. When you reboot, you get a fresh start. We all know that fresh starts feel vital, energized, and efficient. Stopping does not mean inaction. I equate it with eye drops. Respite lubricates your vision.

Respite may be a completely foreign concept to you. If that is so then the following possibilities could stimulate ideas for how you would like to take respite:

1. Meditation, prayer or any mindfulness practice;
2. Meeting with a spiritual mentor;
3. Physical exercise that you enjoy;
4. Spending time in nature;
5. Participating in a support group;
6. Connecting with a trusted friend and sharing your experiences;
7. Enjoying a healthy meal;
8. Attending art events such as exhibits, theater, dance, concerts or film perhaps with others whose interests you share;
9. Receiving massage or other healing treatment;
10. Reading wonderful books;
11. Attending a retreat or workshop ;
12. Researching organizations and community resources for yourself and your family;
13. Humor;
14. Gardening; and
15. Simply being present to yourself.

The next two chapters introduce you to specific practices that serve as respite. Chapter Nine points you towards organizations with a respite orientation. Review the concept of the Caregiver Steward's need for regeneration at the end of Chapter One to underscore your awareness of the core values of honoring your own health and wellbeing.

Few can ready you for the emotions that may surface during respite. War fuses feelings together so that they are indistinguishable from each other. This is especially true for those who provide care because they are bound to being listeners. Respite is a space that allows compacted feelings to breathe. This can either be through expression or relaxation, such as enjoying a good comedy or having a massage. Once you feel you have more room inside yourself, it is easier to understand and articulate your experiences and communicate your needs, even to yourself.

Respite creates the conditions that allow the mind and body to unravel from the stressors of caregiving. Removed from the caregiving environment, the care provider feels themselves to be who they are rather than solely a caregiver. All the senses are reshuffled during respite. Nothing qualifies as sensory overload as thoroughly as the conditions of war brought home. Sensory reintegration is what happens during respite.

As we look at the characteristics of creating respite it is clear that these are the antithesis of the hypervigilant conditions of war and combat that soldiers bring home with them and that they introduce into their environments. The state of respite clarifies for the caregiver that he or she is not at war. The greatest evidence for this is that there is space for respite. You are allowed to stop.

The point here is that respite creates the opportunity for the caregiver's nervous system to be differentiated from that of the veteran. This differentiation is the antidote to burnout. It allows for the cultivation of Resilient Empathy. Differentiation is the alternative to contamination by the environment that war brings home.

Community and Respite

"Recovery is a matter of shared moral engagement."
☐ Nancy Sherman[2]

Asking for help allows others to participate in your healing and the healing of your family. This is a gift to them. In her book, *Afterwar*, Nancy Sherman advocates for a dialogue between civilians and the families of veterans, as well as with veterans themselves, as a way to manifest individual and global healing of the wounds of war. Asking civilians in your community to co-participate so that you can receive respite generates such dialogue.

Asking for help is also an act of faith in humanity. If you invite someone to cover the time and the tasks that will allow you to have respite, whether this is a family member or people from your church or community, you open the door to new relationships and unpredictable experiences. Eileen McKinley's experience in Chapter Three illustrates this. Eileen's decision to ask for help created a previously unimagined and optimistic future for her family. The benefits reverberated for years to come. This is what can happen when you move away from self-sabotage.

Finally, asking for help is a ritual of regeneration in itself. When veterans and their families invite individual civilians and civilian organizations to share their burden of recovery, a collective moral responsibility is more evenly distributed. This salves the moral wounds of war for everyone in a just and appropriate manner. Beyond anger and beyond blame, all of us, civilian and military alike, citizen and politico, are here together living with what happens when war comes home. Let's roll up our sleeves and do the work together to restore health for soldiers and for their families. It is an act of integrity for caregivers to ask for help in their communities and for them to take respite as a result of that help.

Some of the organizations I mention in Chapter Nine were created to allow veterans, family members and caregivers to take respite. Many of these were established by those who know through their first-hand experience that respite is a necessity. These portray a variety of respite options, including opportunities for families as a whole to take respite together. The REST House model in Chapter Ten includes respite for family members by sharing the burden of care. True transition necessitates a provision for respite for care-givers.

The Seven Steps of Respite

Following these seven steps launches a lifestyle that incorporates respite. All of us return to the sequence, beginning with the first step, multiple times.

1. Unmask and release guilt and shame;
2. Realize that the mountain of caregiving demands is endless and will always lead to overwhelm. Therefore, trying relentlessly to meet those demands in order to take respite is an impossible order of priorities. Stop before you are exhausted and take respite;
3. Reach out for help from trusted others to take over caregiving for you so that respite is possible;

4. Schedule your respite options;
5. Experience respite;
6. Repeat the options that provide satisfying respite and remain open to new ways of taking respite; and
7. Establish an ongoing schedule so that respite is a committed aspect of your lifestyle.

In the light of the definition I propose, respite is whatever allows you to reconfigure and recalibrate your situation in relationship to how war has come home in your life. It is when we see the conditions in our lives in a new way that resiliency is born. Respite is an innate component of accepting that war has come home and we have to do something about that.

In the first section of this book I have described the mechanisms with which war comes home and the impacts of those mechanisms on the families of veterans. Section Two is about how we move forward, utilizing empowered feelings, health and creativity. War reshapes us, but we remain whole. Respite opens us to this realization.

Chapter 6 Notes

1. Milliken, C. S., et al (2007) Longitudinal Assessment of Mental Health Problems among Active and Reserve Component Soldiers returning from the Iraq War. *Journal of the American Medical Association.* Nov.14; 298(18):2141 – 2148.

2. Sherman, N. (2015) *Afterwar: Healing the Moral Wounds of Our Soldiers.* New York: Oxford University Press.

Chapter Seven

Creating Your Life: Creative Strategies for the Families of Veterans

"Writing brings higher brain frequencies back into service rather than allowing the brain and body to remain in fight or flight mode."
☐ Ron Capps, Originator of Veterans Writing Project[1]

What saved me as I grew up in the shadow of my father's combat shock was my ability to express myself in safe ways. As a young child this expression was internalized, but once I was able to write this outlet became my constant ally. It has endured as a resource. Writing can be a superb vehicle for cutting through chaos. It evokes focus, perspective, and meaning. Writing tools tend to be readily available. A writing practice, if prioritized, creates a shelter of time and space. Writing is a path to differentiation and differentiation is the key to liberation from Secondary Traumatization.

Any expressive undertaking that allows you to see yourself and your experience more objectively fuels differentiation. The visual arts, for instance, can function this way. Whatever releases feeling leads to the potential for differentiation. Music, movement, and singing will serve this purpose. I emphasize writing in this chapter because it is the tool that I have used predominantly and it has served me well. You can, however, translate the exercises that I have developed for you in this chapter to other arts. For instance, instead of spontaneous and purposeful writing you can try spontaneous and purposeful painting.

While there are a few writing programs for veterans that are exemplary, like the Veterans Writing Project, to my knowledge, a parallel program of equal scope for partners and family members has not yet developed . I do my best to inspire one in these pages. The simple act of writing is a stress reliever and it is completely free. Educational levels are irrelevant. I can tell you from my own personal experience that giving yourself permission to write is a direct route to reclaiming your selfhood from what happens when war comes home.

This chapter launches a writing program for its readers. It offers strategies, exercises and writing templates. Use them as an overall approach to creative expression. The purpose is to celebrate the truth that the telling of our stories, in whatever form feels natural, breaks the spell of trauma. The renowned writer Laura Hildebrand, author of one of the greatest books about surviving the horrors of war, *Unbroken*, says about her father's war experiences, "I always wanted to understand how hard it must have been for him but he never talked about it. He never discussed the emotional consequences."[2] Hildebrand met another soldier, one who this time was willing and able to talk. His name was Louis Zamperini. She dispelled her father's mysterious silence by artfully communicating the trials of a World War warrior who wanted to keep no secrets.

When your voice is heard in whatever form you chose, first by yourself and then perhaps by others you trust, an act of magic is performed. You emerge from hiding as a distinct individual. You come into focus. This is the essence of empowerment. It is reclamation. If, however, you have never written or expressed yourself creatively before, or if it has been a long time since you have considered creative expression that is for and about yourself, you may not know how to begin. Read on to jump-start your new beginning.

How to Begin?

"Consciousness comes from a wholehearted surrender to the moment."
☐ Fr. Richard Rohr[3]

Writing, or any expressive medium, is a path to clarity. If you have no prior experience with creative expression you may feel intimidated at the suggestion of doing it. Please know that the creative experience is, at its core, always simple and accessible. Ignore the voices that tell you otherwise. You start with where you are. Here are some basic first steps.

1. Find a time and a place to write or paint, draw or make your chosen form of music. Finding this time and place may prove to be your greatest challenge. Nevertheless, I assure you that both are available to you. You have to choose and prioritize them.
2. Determine what is most physically and emotionally comfortable for you in terms of how you want to express yourself. As an example, if writing is your medium, determine whether you want to write with a pen in a notebook, or do you prefer to use your computer or another device? You can speak into a recording application or use a voice command for your computer, notebook or phone.
3. Assure that you have adequate lighting so that you can sit and write (or paint or draw or write songs) at ease. I suggest eliminating the presence of all technology and any other distractions.
4. Create safety, confidentiality and containment for yourself.
5. Establish the ambience that is pleasing to you. Do not fuss over this. It should be a simple, convenient arrangement. You can also create this outside the home if necessary. Writers can find a place at a library or in a café. Artists can paint and draw outdoors. Movement is an expressive medium that serves me as well as writing and often in combination with writing. I have rented dance studios for an hour or two at a time. The rent was surprisingly affordable and the feeling of spaciousness was uplifting and inspiring. The hardest part was giving

myself permission to rent the studio and making sure that I went there.

Two seemingly paradoxical states are engaged for your creative time. These are:

1.   Spontaneity; and
2.   Purpose.

Spontaneity

Allow the flood of impressions that have welled up inside you to pour out onto the page, the computer, the easel or the dance floor. The greatest healing comes from not resisting what is. Your expression can be solely for your own eyes. Let it be raw, uncensored, unstructured free flow. Grammar, spelling, punctuation and sentence structure are irrelevant, as are lyrical sounds or representational art. This is your space and your time. Lean into it with the full weight of your truth. The more you express, the lighter you will feel.

Spontaneous creativity allows your internal life to breathe deeply. It is an antidote to depression. Depression and despair are fed by accumulations of negative self-talk and the suppression of authenticity. Spontaneous expression is Bearing Witness to you. It is like a torch lighting a wide span, exposing and illuminating the way forward.

Spontaneous creativity provides the source material for the purposeful expression that can come later, but it is worthwhile unto itself. It is permission to download unfiltered impressions and be present to them. When you see into the mirror of your own world without shame or blame you give yourself the opportunity to go beyond your circumstances.

Even though spontaneous expression is, by definition, unrestricted, it does flourish with a few structures. The instruction is simply that you put pen to paper, if writing is your medium, and write – without stopping, without interrupting your flow, without correcting yourself. You just keep going for a proscribed period of time that you establish for yourself. Please note that if this spontaneous approach does not appeal to you, you can skip this section and go directly to a more purposeful approach or find an alternate structure of your own. The principle here is to provide an avenue for individuation so that you can be free of Secondary Traumatization. Choose the medium that suits you best. The Centering suggestions that follow support you regardless of whether you are creating spontaneously, with purpose, or neither, having taken your own direction with your expression. I am going to frame these steps for the writing experience but feel free to translate them for your chosen form of expression. Just substitute your art form for the word "writing" wherever you see it.

1. Preface your Spontaneous Writing with centering;
2. Do your Spontaneous Writing for the amount of time that feels right to you. I suggest starting with ten or fifteen minutes. The time frame is adjustable as you become more at ease and familiar with this process; and
3. End your Spontaneous Writing interval with another centering experience.

Centering helps you become fluid and open before and as you write, and it helps you to relax when you are done. It also helps to define the entry into and the exit out of this focus. It is a marker. If any of the templates I provide do not suit you, find others. You could, for instance, use meditation or prayer.

Writing is a synthesizing process. It awakens concentration and focus. It utilizes multiple brain centers simultaneously and is thereby integrative. This makes it the perfect expressive medium for people who live in the midst of ongoing stress, such as when war comes home. Writing is an incredibly easy way to de-fog the haze of the chaos and Secondary Traumatization that war brings home. It is a breath of clean, fresh air. Parents can learn how to encourage their children at various ages to write. They can also learn structures for writing with them. These templates are in my book, *New Frontiers in Sensory Integration*.[4]

Centering and Spontaneous Writing Exercises
#1: Grounded Writing

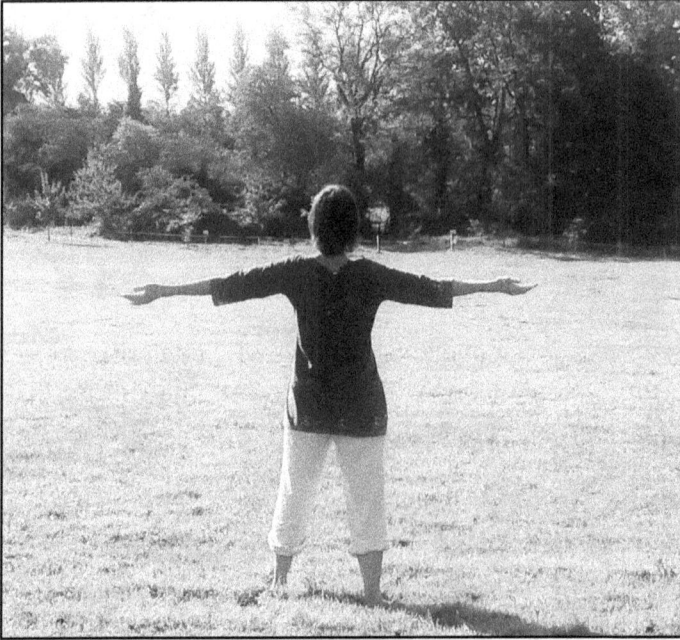

Figure 7.1

Start in a comfortable stance in your writing space, wherever that may be. Let the soles of your feet touch the ground. Close your eyes. Put your attention on the area just under the mound of your big toes on the soles of your feet. This is Site #6 in the applied touch system that is described in Chapter Eight. The function of this site is to provide balance.

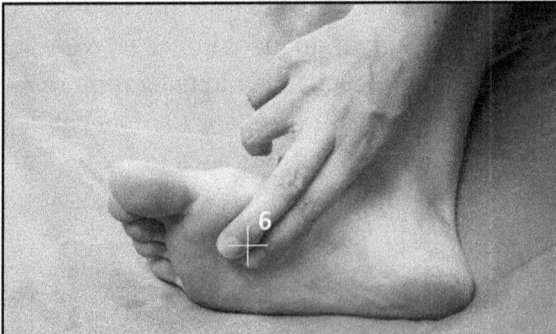

Figure 7.2

Imagine that a root, like the root of a tree, is growing from that place into the earth. Let that root that connects you to the earth be strong and pulsing with life. Feel it supporting and sustaining you. Breathe deeply and fully as you feel this connection. When it is solid, open your eyes and write spontaneously. Let the writing pour forth of its own accord. If you feel stuck, keep writing. You can repeat the most recent sentence or any statement but as your hands move across the page new language will eventually emerge. Follow your own rhythms. Let your writing go wherever it wants to go. It does not have to make sense. Just keep writing for at least ten or fifteen minutes.

#2: Expansive Writing

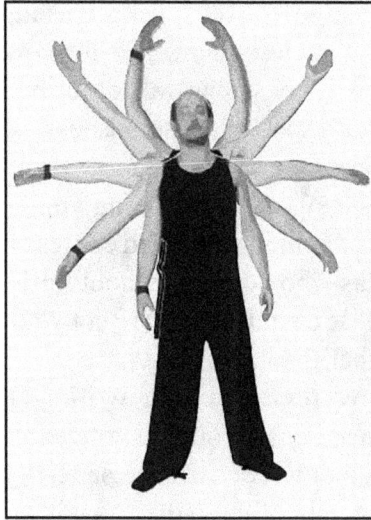

Figure 7.3

This exercise infuses your writing with power and vitality. It is useful when you need to cut through distractions and just do it! Stand in your writing space with your feet hip-width apart. Bring your arms above your head and turn the palms outward. Push through the center of your palms as you allow your arms to descend to your sides slowly. You are making space for yourself. Your chest will open naturally as you do this, allowing you to breathe more fully as you lower your arms. Do this several times.

You can close your eyes. Visualize yourself pushing away anything that interferes with the space you are making for yourself. When you have done this movement enough times so that you feel you have created your space internally as well as externally, sit down and write spontaneously. When you have written for 10-15 minutes, or for the time that feels right for your experience, allow yourself to sit quietly for a few moments, focusing on your breath. You can return to the visualization of the area on the soles of your feet, under the mound of the big toes (#6) that awakens your sense of being rooted, held by the earth, and supported. Feel the relief. You have cleared a trail for yourself into the unknown.

Reviewing Your Spontaneous Writing

You may choose to collect several episodes of spontaneous writing before you review them. For the review, cultivate the attitude of Bearing Witness that was described in Chapter Two. Bearing Wtiness, as a state of consciousness, is your greatest ally in the writing process.

When you first review your writing you are seeing yourself through the prism of your unrestrained expression. You are getting to know yourself as who you are without limitation, obligations, duties or agendas. Be clear that you are not yet editing. Your focus is on listening rather than rewriting.

After you have reviewed your writing from this listening and Bearing Witness stance you will notice that there are themes within your spontaneity. You will see patterns of expression and statements of need. Out of these themes will arise the next phase of Purposeful Writing. This phase arises organically from the rich soil of your Spontaneous Writing. You are leaning into the unknown whenever you write spontaneously; you are a trail blazer when you review your writing and you are pressing the restart button in your brain when you write with purpose.

Purposeful Writing

As you review your collection of spontaneous writings, keep a separate notebook handy. This notebook will contain what you distill from the rich raw ecology of your Spontaneous Writing. In the review process you extract your own guidance. The first step is to itemize the themes you identify. List these themes in the second notebook, or in another computer file. The themes will stand out to you because they are reiterated; some may surprise you.

Examples of possible themes might be:

1. Relational struggles;
2. Dreams;
3. Recurrent memories;
4. Fears;
5. Past traumas;
6. Other people who have played significant roles in your life;
7. Parenting questions;
8. Spiritual questions;
9. Health issues or concerns;
10. Intrusive imagery;
11. Guilt;
12. Grief;
13. Finances;
14. Developmental threshold experiences (for instance, things that happened during adolescence);
15. Frustrations; and
16. Sexuality.

The themes are yours. They evolve out of the specific dynamics of your life and who you really are. They will jump out to meet you from the pages of your Spontaneous Writing. I have provided examples but your themes cannot be predicted.

Select one of these themes and use it as a title for a separate page in your Spontaneous Writing notebook or file. Write spontaneously about this theme. You can do this for each or for as many of the selected themes as you are drawn to explore. In this way you are beginning to sort through the overload from the shock that your body has stored since the moment that war came home. This moment likely preceded when a veteran returned; it may have originated with deployment or preparing for deployment. You become your own commentator for how you got lost in the forest of overload. You also become a torchbearer for yourself by illuminating the way out of the dense foliage of war brought home.

Purposeful Writing: Using Your Two Notebooks

You now have two notebooks or two files on your computer. One contains Spontaneous Writing. The other contains the major themes you have identified. This is your Purposeful Writing notebook. The list of themes represent the options you have identified for your Purposeful Writing. Select one of the themes and review your Spontaneous Writing about it from the perspective of Bearing Witness. You can now write about your chosen theme purposefully. Title a blank page in your Purposeful Writing notebook or open and name a new document on your computer. You are now ready to write with purpose.

You take a giant step in the direction of greater wellbeing and overall health when you extract themes from your life and address them with purpose, particularly after you have fleshed out all the feelings in these themes through Spontaneous Writing. There are many writing formats available for writing purposefully, such as:

1. Write a poem about a theme, encapsulating it in image and metaphor;
2. Write an essay on a theme, seeing yourself delivering your message to an attentive audience;
3. Create a short story or fictionalized character that embodies your theme.

You will be amazed at how your writing talks back to you and affirms that you are your own best guide. Purposeful Writing frees you from passive waiting and empowers you to become proactive. Let's look at examples.

Writing Samples from the Homeland of War

When Rose learned that the partner of a friend had committed suicide, she could barely function. This was the third suicide from her circle of military families. It was only through writing that Rose was able to recover herself and continue being the wonderful mother and wife she wanted to be for her family. She found that poetry was her avenue. After weeks of spontaneous writing in which she felt she was drowning in grief, she emerged with a poem that seemed to spring from nowhere but which synthesized her inner state. Rose felt that inspiration rise within her again when she read the poem out loud to her husband, and then again when she sent it to her email list. Inspiration arose once more when she posted it to a website for veterans. Each time she spoke her truth and claimed her voice she was re-empowered and re-inspired. She was glad to be alive. Here is her poem.

The Distance of the Night

My friends have slipped
Under the dark waters of night,
Men with eyes of fire
And impossible tenderness.
I reach for them across the dimensions
And pull them out fearlessly.
Their tears seep into my flesh.
I will never say good-bye;
I will hunt down their killers;
The one called Feeling Unworthy and the one called Guilty.
Whatever took their breath,
I will hunt it down and remake it over and over
Until their beauty rises again
And their eyes shine
And they tell me what happened to them
And what they know
About the distance of the night.

Rose had written poetry as a teenager but not since then. The experience of writing about loss reminded her of the skills she had when she was younger, and the joy she used to feel when a poem would slip out from her hands and be born, almost fully formed. That was her experience when she wrote "The Distance of the Night," but in fact the poem came from her long immersion in grief and to the ways she had been sensitized to the wounds of war. By becoming a writer again Rose transmuted her grief into advocation and outreach. She crossed over the mourning border into the realm of selfhood. This gave her back the emotional core she remembered and it strengthened her relationships with others, including her husband and her children. Having faced and expressed her confrontation with death and despair, Rose felt the celebration of her choice to live.

Her writing made Rose into someone with a unique and valuable voice. She chose to use that voice when she recognized the emotional undertone that so often pounded in her ears. Rose saw that there was purpose in giving that voice utterance; it lightened burdens, even beyond her own. Grief was not the only theme that emerged as Rose proceeded to investigate her internal world and her writer's vocation. She learned to pay attention to herself and to value how she experienced everything. She gained heightened self-respect. She made time to honor her impressions. As Rose accepted her writer's gift she became a model for others who wanted to speak out about their experiences with war.

The New War Scribes: Essays and Blogs

If you, as the partner or family member of a veteran, begin to write, you will not be alone. I recently counted at least twenty authors who are writing about their experiences when war comes home, and the numbers are growing at a steady clip. Only a few of these were writers before. Combined with the veterans who are writing for their lives, this trend represents the new war scribes, the keepers of the archives of this era of seemingly unending wars. While silence still rules in many homes, in the minority where it does not the word gets out like a clarion call. This is grass roots writing. It is a route to ending lineages of intergenerational traumatic repetition. The technological revolution that keeps us so interconnected is instrumental here. Writers are accessible not only in books but also in blogs and other digital formats that make them easy to read wherever you are.

An excellent example is the writing of Amalie Flynn. Her blogs and books are replete with an honesty that gracefully wakes you up. Her writing could be defined as personal essays; prose memoir pieces that strung together make books. Amalie also writes blogs in an essay format. Her style is poetic. She has developed a format and a rhythm that is purely her own. You can do the same. Here are some examples of Amalie's unique statements.

On Secondary Traumatization:

"War is not over when a country withdraws its troops or a soldier comes home. It slips through the pores of his skin and into the ducts of his house, circulating like blood or heat."

"When deployment is over the bed is full again, war is how two people lay in it, together, but far apart."

On Mobility:

"When I look back now, at our life, together, it lies open, like an atlas. And I can see how it is marked by movement. There is movement over state lines and across oceans and through years, how this is the movement of our marriage.

Our time together, so far, has been seismic.

There has been a geographical lack of commitment. There has been the idea that everything is temporary, everything, even us."

On Healing:

"Things feel different," my husband says.

And we are crossing our front lawn, meeting in the middle, positioned like this, with grass surrounding us like water.

I say yes, and it is getting warmer, but I know he is not talking about weather, but about us, here, in this moment, in this marriage, on this lawn, in front of our house, the house our children are growing up in, with a garden, a garden he planted, growing out back, and our marriage growing inside. He raises his hand up and reaches out, into the thin air, and I reach out and grab it, bringing it back, down, beside me, and into mine.

Because I know what he means, how this is a turn, we are finally starting to face the sun.[5]

You can see how Amalie Flynn has found her own voice and her own style. Her sentence phrasing and use of grammar might not be considered correct by academic standards, but it works for what she wants to convey. We understand and feel her rhythms. They add to our appreciation of how she can convey her own story. Her sharing inspires us to end our own isolation by speaking out.

Other writers from military families use a more declarative voice and fall into a category that I call writer-activists. The best writer-activists speak from their own direct experience to encourage social change. They are compelled to make a difference. As Rosa Parks, one of the most influential social activists of all time said, "I knew what had to be done. Knowing what has to be done does away with fear."[6] Writer activists proliferate during times like this, when the gap between what laws provide and what people really need has widened too far. We know this to be the case for veterans and their families, worldwide. The chasm draws forth voices that would have preferred to remain silent. Courage comes when hearts break.

Here is a short essay written by a mother who felt helpless as she watched her family break under the weight of war brought home. When Courtney began to write, something changed inside her so that she rebounded with enormous energy and a determination to be a good parent to her children, to have fun with them, and to make sure they had a childhood, no matter what. She says it was seeing herself on paper, outside of herself, that made the difference.

A Call to Arms

The corporations that serve the machines of war and the pharmaceutical companies that make medicines; they will not come into my home and take care of my family. War has woven itself into the skin of my children like an ugly tattoo that I cannot erase. The father of my children who once seemed indestructible now is like a diseased child in quarantine.

Trauma is the secret weapon of war. Slow death by trauma steals the smiles off of children's faces. It cracks wide open the hearts of mothers until we have to form our own army of protest, using the shards of our souls as weapons to demand what belongs to us, what our soldiers fought for and what has been taken away from us at home.

I will not be a victim of war in my own house. I have learned to dig deep into my will and my spirit and tired as I might be,

I will rally myself and I will rally others. My children will not forget how to laugh and run and play even if they cannot do these things with their father. When they ask me what happened to their dad, I will tell them the truth. I will say that he gave his all and then there was nothing left. I will say that he has to recover himself and only he can do that. I will say that their dad made a sacrifice for us and that therefore we honor his sacrifice by living a joyful existence. And I will reach out my arms and hug them close so that they can feel my strength.

In 2003, the US National Endowment for the Arts asked soldiers serving in Iraq and Afghanistan, and their families, to contribute whatever they had written about their war related experiences. NEA wanted to create an anthology to document the first hand experiences of those actively serving in these wars. They were flooded with submissions. Most of them were essays.[7] The extreme experiences that are the nature of war and combat dredge the well of creativity and out gushes wisdom, insight, and purpose. "Let your words pour forth from the well of your heart through your hands, and out into the world." This was the beckoning cry of the National Endowment for the Arts. "Hear yourself and let others hear your truths. Have no doubt that this will make a healing difference." This was the motto of the NEA project that produced the anthology *Operation Homecoming.*

The National Endowment project also offered the writers short workshops and mentoring to refine their writing. Writing always demands these two stages: a raw outpouring and careful and clear editing. Anthology editor Andrew Carroll says that he made every effort to retain the authentic voices of the contributors through the editing process. The challenge in the refining process is to intensify rather than lessen passion.

Mind Maps

Mind Maps are a tool for moving from Spontaneous Writing to Purposeful Writing. All you have to do is put your theme in the center of a large piece of paper or just use your notebook page. Colored pens or markers can add to the fun. Out of the encircled theme you draw lines to subsets of your theme, and circle them.

You end up with an array of words in balloon-like circles. This is a visual display of the aspects of your theme. It is a non-linear outline that can point to the development of both the content and the form of what you want to say.

Perhaps you, like Wilson whose essay follows, want to write about how a child experiences life in a military home. You could, as Wilson did, put the words CHILD OF WAR in a large circle in the center of your page. From this balloon you draw lines to other words like NIGHTMARES, CLINGY, SCARED, ANGRY, STUTTERING or HIDING. These words then generate more balloons. Looking at your page you have a sense of whether you will write in prose or poetry; whether you will develop an essay or a children's story. Mind Maps help you put your thoughts into a visual display that takes you to the next step in your writing process. Here's what Wilson's Mind Map looked like.

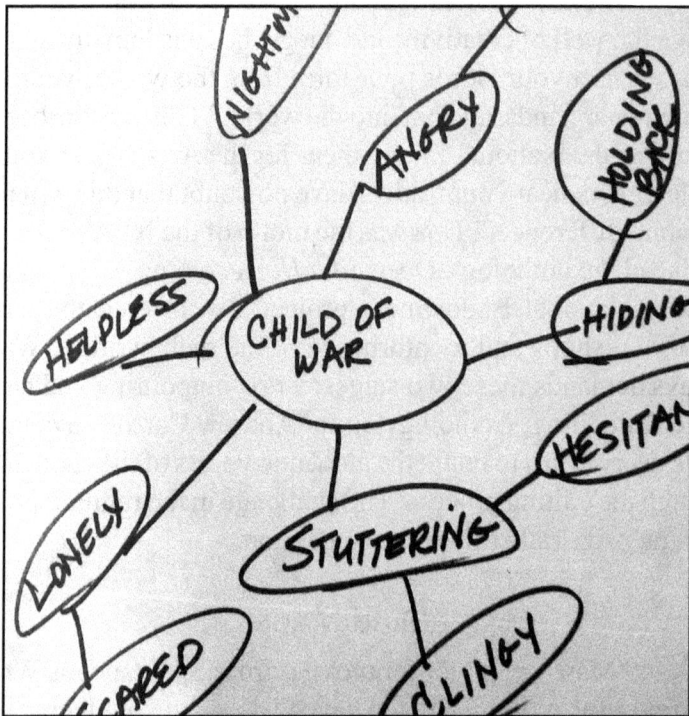

Figure 7.4

This Mind Map was where Wilson started to courageously break down his emotional numbing so that he could connect with his son. Wilson used Mind Maps like this to write the essay that follows and several others.

I See My Son and He Sees Me

When I returned from Iraq I felt like I lived in a cloud. No matter what the weather was outside, I felt overcast. I huddled into myself 24/7. Out of the corner of my eye I could see my son Aaron but I could not really see him. Aaron was a baby when I left and now he is a little boy, almost five years old. I didn't know anything about him really. He was just a moving object outside my range of vision and therefore dangerous. I kept my mouth shut and my eyes averted.

I don't know how this happened but one day, almost a year to the day since my last deployment, the cloud parted and I could see more clearly. It literally seemed as if I got my lenses cleaned even though I do not wear glasses. This came out of nowhere. I don't think I did anything to make it happen. I am grateful to my wife because during this entire time she kept reaching out to me, but she also let me have my space. She is a relationship artist I think. I don't know how she did it because I was no fun to be with but she acted like she was prepared for this somehow. She must have studied something before I came home. That would be like her. She is super smart.

When the cloud parted the first thing I saw was Aaron. I am writing about this so that my buddies and other people who come home to their families might read it and maybe it will not take them as long as it has taken me to see my son. I just saw my son. I saw his innocence. I saw that he wanted me to play with him. I saw his eyes. They were so pure. I saw that he was OK but I also saw that he was in pain. I saw him clinging to things, stuttering, having nightmares, and hiding in corners. But I also saw that in other ways he was OK. He was OK because my wife had been keeping track of him. But he was not OK because he did not know who his dad was.

So I walked up to him and looked in his eyes and I said, "Hey buddy." And he just smiled the biggest smile in the world. And that was really the day that I came home. I saw my son and he saw me, and I was grateful. In that one moment I realized that the whole thing was about Aaron, and other kids like Aaron, boys and girls. So I figured that I better say something about this and I better pay attention to him. I did not want to waste another moment.

Writing for the Children of War

Children are curious about the lives of their parents. All the events that influence the family arouse the interest of the children in that family. In fact, children's brains are shaped by the expectations, degrees of warmth and engagement, and the overall attitudinal states that surround them.[8]

Children feel stress when a family member's behavior is mysterious or disturbing and no one explains why. Depending on their age, children generally do not have the language or the capacity to express their confusion, so it smolders inside them. Children almost always love their parents, and their caring makes them want to help a parent who seems distressed. Again, the child cannot verbalize their impulse to help. If no one notices or engages with the child then ultimately their curiosity finds an answer in self-blame. Family members can prevent this snowball from accumulating trauma by creating demystifying scrapbooks, albums, stories or videos.

Several of the mothers I interviewed in the course of writing this book described to me how they gathered together whatever they could find to portray where the parent who had been deployed had been. They assembled a story that included the geography and the history of that place to give it real meaning and shape. The emphasis was always on providing a context for sharing that individual's experience with a child. When violent events or losses occurred they were de-emphasized or minimized as this was not the focus of the communication. The intention behind this creativity was to give dimension to what was otherwise a blank space in that child's information bank.

This is what Wilson eventually provided for his son Aaron. He created a storybook that contained pictures of his buddies. He talked about himself as a man with friends and with a hard job to do in a place that was hot, dusty and mired in war. He told his son about sleeping outdoors at night and meeting people who spoke another language. He shared the relationships he had with Iraqi families as well as with his army mates. He told Aaron about the children he met who could have been Aaron's peers. He gave those children names. He included in his story how he felt when he heard about Aaron's adventures in his world, like riding a tricycle or starting pre-school and making friends. Thus Wilson slowed down his own nervous system and answered his son's unvoiced questions. Sometimes what it takes to resolve trauma is to see it through the eyes of a child.

The Healing Powers of Language

In fiction and in film war has been characterized predominantly from the male soldier's point of view. Stereotypes abound. Soldiers are alienated, self-destructive, isolated, violent, bombastic or confused. Family members are shocked, passive, struggling, victimized, or supportive and self-effacing. These portrayals etch their way into consciousness, determining how we regard, or disregard, the families of veterans. This makes the families of veterans anonymous. It is as if individual characteristics are stripped away. When family members write to share their true experiences of how war comes home, those stereotypes dissolve.

Essays, poems, children's stories, scrapbook documentation and reflections are just some of the writing forms available to us. Another option is writing creatively; allowing the magical play of the imagination to find its way into language to reveal, through fictionalized characters, the characteristics of war brought home. Writing fiction, whether short stories, novellas or novels, is another way to allow writing to be an antidote to Secondary Traumatization.

Toni Morrison, for instance, tells the fictional story of Korean War veteran Frank Money and his sister Cee who are separated by war. When the war ends Frank wanders America, stunned by his disconnected mind, his inability to focus, his hauntings, and his refusal to go home. Only his sister's life threatening illness arouses his motivation and he returns to help her. Standing in a field, at the base of a tree that has been cleft by lightening but that is still miraculously alive, Frank experiences a rite of passage. This is his ritual of homecoming. His internal experience is recorded as a poem within the novel.

> *I stood there a long while, staring at that tree.*
> *It looked so strong.*
> *So beautiful.*
> *Hurt right down the middle*
> *But alive and well.*
> *Cee touched my shoulder*
> *Lightly.*
> *Frank?*
> *Yes?*
> *Come on brother. Let's go home.*[9]

The power of expression to relieve stress and to honor our humanity is extraordinary. In fact, some believe that expression, even more than meditation or relaxation, is the most potent form of recovery from trauma. Whatever art form magnetizes you, my admonition is to not withhold expression. Let nothing stop you from enjoying your innate creativity as an antidote to how war comes home.

Chapter 7 Notes

1. Capps, R. US Army and Foreign Service veteran. Director of the Veterans Writing Project. This is a non-profit organization, based in Washington DC, that provides no-cost writing seminars and workshops for veterans.

2. Hildebrand, L. (2014). Taken from an interview with Wil S. Hylton 'The Unbreakable Laura Hildebrand' in the New York Times, Sunday Magazine, Dec. 18th; pg MM36.

3. Rohr, Fr R. (2008) To Be Awake is to Live in the Present. Collection of Homolies 2008.

4. Mines, S. (2014) *New Frontiers in Sensory Integration: Limbic Stimulation, Authentic Relationship and a Multi-Disciplinary Treatment Design.* Pgs 118-126. Stillwater, OK: New Forums Press

5. Flynn, A. (2013) These statements are taken from Amalie's blog Wife and War: The Memoir. Rhode Island, USA. www.wifeandwar.wordpress.com

6. Parks, R, L., Reed, G. J. (1994) *Quiet Strength: The Faith, the Hope, and the Heart of a Woman who changed the Nation.* MI: Zondervan Publishing House.

7. Carroll, A. (2006) *Operation Homecoming: Iraq, Afghanistan, and the Home Front, in the Words of US Troops and Their Families.* New York: Random House.

8. Proceedings of the US National Academy of Sciences, July 20, 2015: Researchers from Princeton University, the University of Rochester and the University of South Carolina found that babies as young as 5 months old respond by modulating their brains when learning expectations are directed at them, regardless of whether or not there are any actions taken in association with those expectations. This research, focused entirely on infants, demonstrates the interactive, relational nature of the learning dynamic.

9. Morrison, T. (2012) *Home.* New York: Random House

Chapter Eight

Your Hands Heal: Applied Touch for the Invisible Wounds of War

It was because of war that I met the woman who brought healing home to me. While my father was in combat in Europe, Mariko Iino was placed in an internment camp in the United States. As I developed in the care of a distraught mother, an adolescent Mariko struggled with rage in a dusty, crowded shed where her family, once prosperous and refined, was forced to live. When her camp was liberated, Mariko, a young woman by then, declared she would leave America to live forever in her homeland in Japan. Not long after her arrival in Japan Mariko met a man who changed her heart, her nervous system and her life. Jiro Murai, a revered healing master, taught her an applied touch practice that transformed her rage into compassion. Thirty years later I met Mariko, who by then was called Mary, in Northern California, and she transmitted that same gift to me. Like Mary at the time she met Jiro Murai, I too was at a turning point.

Mary taught me an approach to healing that shakes trauma from the nervous system with such ease that it is like shaking out a blanket. The phrase "coming home" gained new meaning when I practiced what Mary taught me. I came home to the health and vitality that is my birthright. I was also able to find my ground while adjusting to a new life as a single mother with my little daughter in a place that was completely new to us. Mary provided my transition medicine.

Given how the transmission of this healing wisdom from Jiro Murai to Mary arose from war, it is fitting that it be offered back to the families of war. I provide the applications of this art that are the most suited to the families of veterans in this book. If we know that war comes home, then we also deserve to know that healing comes home.

When I first met Mary I was a single working mother trying to earn a decent living while simultaneously being both mother and father to my child. I could not afford expensive therapies. Learning the healing art that Mary offered empowered me to climb out of self-doubt and feel capable and competent under trying circumstances. The system, which I call Jin Shin TARA, to honor Mary's heritage of Jin Shin and the TARA (Tools for Awakening Resources and Awareness) Approach I developed, makes a difference every time I use it. Now over thirty-five years later, I still rely on it to help me overcome any lingering insecurities, physical illnesses, spiritual dilemmas and life crises. I use it for my children and my grandchildren. It has supported my husband in recovering admirably from catastrophic accidents and life-threatening conditions. It has made it possible for one of my children to be free of the consequences of a cranial anomaly and avoid surgeries. The system has now been tested in numerous clinical trials and it is consistently shown to be of benefit for conditions as complex as Traumatic Brain Injury, autism, stroke and aphasia.[1,2,3,4,5,6]

The applications intervene in how the nervous system reacts. They decondition habituated behaviors. The felt sense of being different internally and therefore capable of responding in new ways is thoroughly empowering, liberating and inspirational. Once experienced, there is no turning back. The remarkable breakthrough for me was learning first hand that I could invite the innate healing response in my body to take over through my own touch.

I cannot say that these applications are a panacea, or that they are curative for the myriad ways in which war comes home. I can confidently say, however, that they will help, in some way, everyone who uses them, particularly if they are used consistently. There are no contraindications and you can do no harm. The applications are completely safe to use for and with children. My book, *New Frontiers in Sensory Integration*, provides protocols for neurodiverse children and youth with sensory and learning challenges using this applied touch system.[7]

I have learned not to predict how anyone will respond to these applications. This is because I have been repeatedly surprised when someone who I thought would be skeptical or resistant instead reported pain relief, rejuvenation, and a diminution of troubling, chronic symptoms. Therefore I have become increasingly more generous in not only offering the treatments but also in my confidence that the most simple interventions, such as those that I present here, can make a real difference.

While the practices I suggest in this book are primarily for the partners and family members of wounded warriors, they can also be used by veterans themselves, as well as by the therapists who serve them and who can recommend these interventions. The applications will not contradict a physician's care, and they are not intended to replace it. This is an integrative medicine and collaborates with all other interventions in a positive way.

The functional mechanism of Jin Shin TARA is human bioelectricity. We know that bioelectricity exists because it is detected in imaging technologies like CAT scans, electrocardiograms and MRI's, all of which measure bioelectricity for diagnostic purposes. Jin Shin was developed long before such instruments existed. It uses human touch to measure bioelectrical frequencies. Acupuncture employs a similar diagnostic process in pulse reading. The pulse that is read is a bioelectrical rhythm. In Jin Shin TARA we touch prescribed areas of the body to first read and then improve bioelectrical conductivity. When we hold two areas in combination and feel that their bioelectrical pulsations are synchronized, then we know that we have stabilized or balanced that frequency. Some people encounter difficulty in feeling pulsation or bioelectrical rhythms. Sensitivity often improves with practice, but even if it does not, there are other indicators that can be used to substitute for pulse reading. Changes in breathing or subtle variations in skin tone or state of mind can be observed to reveal how the nervous system is coming into balance.

A Map of Hope

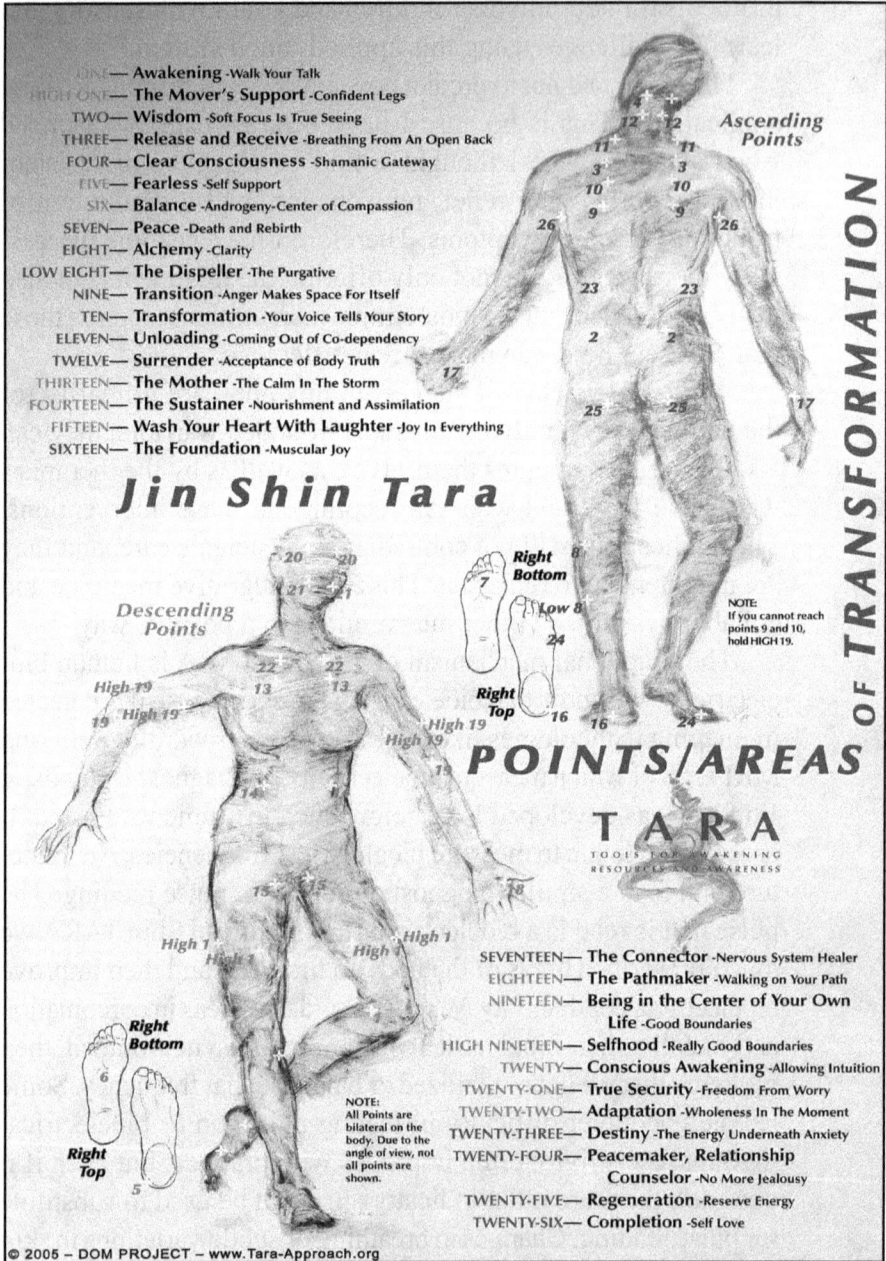

ONE— **Awakening** -Walk Your Talk
HIGH ONE— **The Mover's Support** -Confident Legs
TWO— **Wisdom** -Soft Focus Is True Seeing
THREE— **Release and Receive** -Breathing From An Open Back
FOUR— **Clear Consciousness** -Shamanic Gateway
FIVE— **Fearless** -Self Support
SIX— **Balance** -Androgeny-Center of Compassion
SEVEN— **Peace** -Death and Rebirth
EIGHT— **Alchemy** -Clarity
LOW EIGHT— **The Dispeller** -The Purgative
NINE— **Transition** -Anger Makes Space For Itself
TEN— **Transformation** -Your Voice Tells Your Story
ELEVEN— **Unloading** -Coming Out of Co-dependency
TWELVE— **Surrender** -Acceptance of Body Truth
THIRTEEN— **The Mother** -The Calm In The Storm
FOURTEEN— **The Sustainer** -Nourishment and Assimilation
FIFTEEN— **Wash Your Heart With Laughter** -Joy In Everything
SIXTEEN— **The Foundation** -Muscular Joy

Jin Shin Tara

Ascending Points

Descending Points

Right Bottom

Right Top

NOTE:
If you cannot reach points 9 and 10, hold HIGH 19.

POINTS/AREAS

OF *TRANSFORMATION*

T A R A
TOOLS FOR AWAKENING
RESOURCES AND AWARENESS

Right Bottom

Right Top

NOTE:
All Points are bilateral on the body. Due to the angle of view, not all points are shown.

SEVENTEEN— **The Connector** -Nervous System Healer
EIGHTEEN— **The Pathmaker** -Walking on Your Path
NINETEEN— **Being in the Center of Your Own Life** -Good Boundaries
HIGH NINETEEN— **Selfhood** -Really Good Boundaries
TWENTY— **Conscious Awakening** -Allowing Intuition
TWENTY-ONE— **True Security** -Freedom From Worry
TWENTY-TWO— **Adaptation** -Wholeness In The Moment
TWENTY-THREE— **Destiny** -The Energy Underneath Anxiety
TWENTY-FOUR— **Peacemaker, Relationship Counselor** -No More Jealousy
TWENTY-FIVE— **Regeneration** -Reserve Energy
TWENTY-SIX— **Completion** -Self Love

© 2005 – DOM PROJECT – www.Tara-Approach.org

Figure 8.1

The areas we hold are depicted on this chart as areas of transformation. I call them the Sacred Sites of the Body. They are centers for specific mind-body functions. The map is quite simple, with only 26 basic areas. This makes it easy to use and remember, like the 26 letters of the alphabet. I use the word "areas" to emphasize that you are not being asked to hold a point or a precise position. Rather these centers are fields with at least a four inch radius. This is one of the reasons why you cannot make an error by holding the "wrong" area. As long as you are within the energetic field of the site, then your touch is positive and effective in stimulating and balancing the current there.

You can use any part of your hand or fingers to hold the sites. You can also use either your right or your left hand to hold the sites. The key is to be relaxed and comfortable. Sometimes you may use self-care in a public place and will want to be discreet. This is easy to do. You will see this in the examples that follow.

Look at the map and review where the sites are and their names. I have framed the names to reflect the primary functions of the sites. The combinations of sites that I provide for specific protocols are developed from the theoretical templates that Mary taught and that she learned from Jiro Murai. The applications that follow are basic. They do not utilize all of the sites. My intention is to provide a sampler of how to harmlessly and gently engage with the nervous system. I hope that my readers will experiment by combining the sites freely. I have great confidence in the positive outcomes that are inevitable from using this system. There is a treasury of specific applications that I am eager to share with the families of veterans so those who want more should not hesitate to contact me.

The Art of Holding Yourself

Most of the sites on the body can be reached easily for self-care. The ones that appear more challenging to reach, such as those on the back, can be replaced by holding the sites that are in front of them. For instance, you can hold Site #13 on the chest if you cannot reach Site #9 on the back. Massaging, tapping or rubbing the areas is not recommended. Light touch is fine. You can use the palm of your hand to encompass an entire area if you prefer that to holding the site with one or two fingers. This is a holding practice that gives you the gift of being with yourself rather than doing something to yourself.

Bioeectrical currents run throughout the body and are conducted by skin. When holding the sites you are likely to feel a pulsation arising from them. This is bioelectrical current. If you do not detect a current you may, instead, feel a change in temperature or another sensation. The pulse, if you feel it, is different from blood pulse because of its variability. It is the balancing of this pulsation that harmonizes the sites. You will feel the balance in your fingertips and you will also notice shifts in your body. Do not be concerned if the pulse is not apparent to you. Focus on the other sensations, such as a deepening of the breath or a feeling of ease, to validate your effectiveness. People often try too hard to feel the pulse and are discouraged when they assume they do not. This is not a practice of efforting so follow the path of least resistance and enjoy your experience. Be curious about it rather than critical.

A good place to begin exploring is with #1.

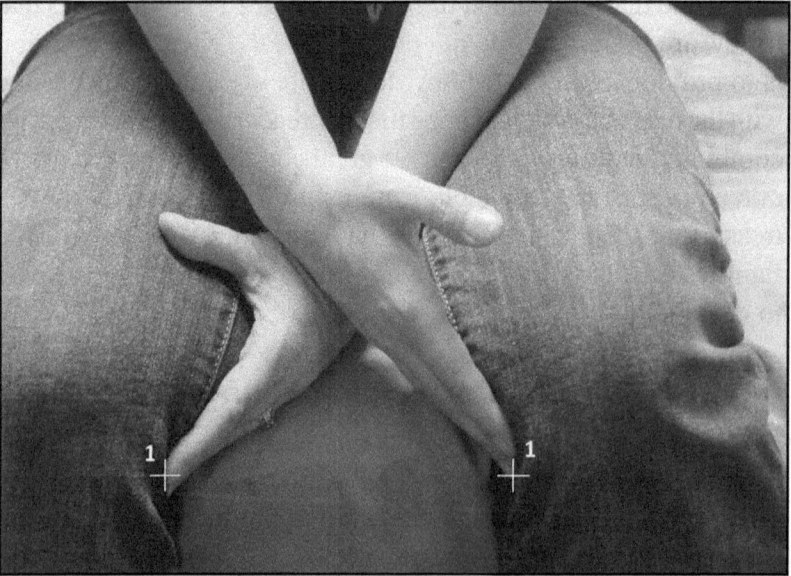

Figure 8.2

Try holding this position inside the knee. Put your fingertips on the bilateral sites in any way that is comfortable for you. It might be best to access these sites from a seated position. You can cross your hands if that improves your feeling of being at ease, as depicted in Figure 8.2, but that is not required. Notice the quality of your own contact. This site is sometimes said to have a "grounding" influence. This means that it helps to calm the mind and the body, allowing you to feel "rooted" or connected to the earth. This makes holding #1 helpful for people with head injuries because it opens an alternate neuronal pathway of calm and ease when they are upset. Partners and family members can hold this site on themselves so that their reactions to the soldier's behavior are calmed. This lessens the likelihood of accelerating a problematic situation.

Living with someone with TBI demands an evolution in awareness. Unless someone is alerted to how to maintain stability, home dynamics can spin out of control. Holding Sacred Site #1 slows everything down. If reaching it is difficult for any reason, there is an alternate approach. This is called High One. Then make these changes so that this reads: You contact High One in two positions on the mid-thigh as shown in Figure 8.3. Crossing your hands is not necessary but it is an option if that is most comfortable for you.

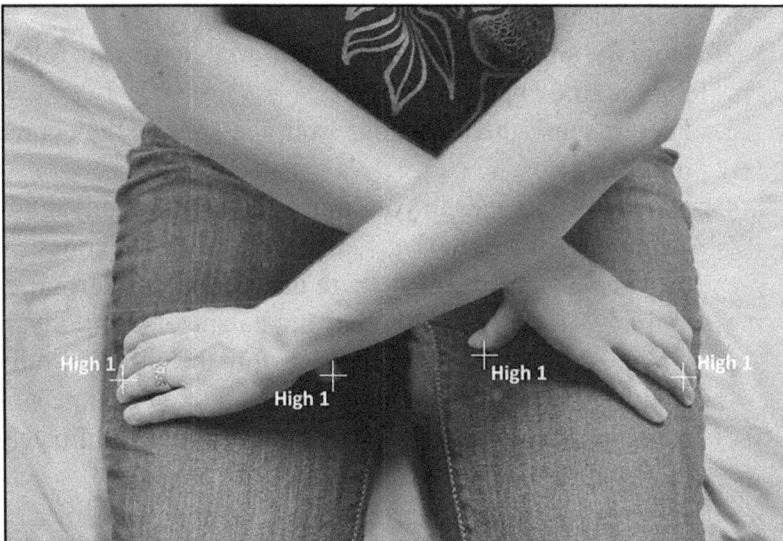

Figure 8.3

115

High One and Site #1 also send supportive bioelectrical current to the knee structures, including the joints, ligaments and tendons. This helps balance and movement, both of which are sometimes weakened as a result of head injuries. These benefits extend to an emotional sense of feeling connected and present. You will likely notice that you are breathing more deeply when you hold these areas. Try it! You may notice other benefits as well since each of the sites performs multiple functions.

Noticing the shifts in your sensation and throughout your body is a ritual of regeneration when you hold these areas. You can use the applications here even in the midst of stressful circumstances. You do not have to isolate yourself. I use the practices that I provide in these pages to address all the challenges of my life. If I am nervous about speaking in public; if I feel congested; if I am agitated, I discreetly hold the appropriate sites on my body and inevitably I arrive at a more peaceful, clearer, centered place. Then I can move forward with consciousness and face the obstacle, the day, the situation or the person that appeared to be challenging.

Here are the basic steps for using this applied touch system to offer new options to your mind and your body.

1. Identify the sites you want to hold using the map of the body and the information in this chapter;
2. Hold the sites in a way that is comfortable for you, relaxing into the experience;
3. Feel or sense the pulsations from the sites as they come into balance;
4. Notice the changes in your mind and in your body; and
5. Remove your hands when you feel the process is complete or whenever you like, as there is no harm done from remaining on the sites after they are balanced. Similarly, if you need to remove your hands before the sites feel fully balanced, no harm is done either. You open channels of bioelectricity whenever you contact these sites. Ultimately the repetition of contact will stimulate balance.

The entire practice of using applied touch is a form of active mindfulness. If you think these fundamentals require a sensitivity and subtlety that is hard to imagine in your busy, chaotic life, think again. Sometimes the most agitated people are the ones who can tune in the most deeply to the rhythms of energy. Feel free to experiment with contacting all the sites on the map. Mary Iino Burmeister said, "You are the artist," when encouraging others to use the full palette of these sites.

An Index for Individuation

For family members and veterans who feel enveloped by trauma it seems impossible to individuate from it. Intrusive imagery, nightmares, explosions of rage and frustration, or an overwhelming need to withdraw occur on their own, apparently without an identified choice to initiate them. It is in fact because we are steeping in an environment of trauma that this is so. We have not found a way to differentiate ourselves from it. It is the trauma talking and not our essential selves. Your discerning and intelligent self is lost in the downpour of trauma and cannot see its way clear to be in charge. It is like trying to drive in a blizzard when your windshield wipers are broken. This is the nature of both the primary and the secondary traumatization that afflicts veterans and their family members.

The self-care practices that follow are focused on differentiating from the ways that combat trauma infects our homes. I have selected a few of the most common experiences. Though these practices appear elementary, they are nevertheless revelatory. After more than thirty years of using this system I find that the most basic practices evoke the greatest relief.

Activation and Anxiety

Understanding the mechanics of anxiety is one way to come out of it. When we understand something it has less power to control us. A different part of the brain goes into action as soon as we begin learning. The executive brain becomes engaged and it can curtail the instinctual, knee-jerk responses that generate anxiety. This is why education is a golden key to unlock the patterns of intergenerational traumatic repetition when war comes home. Without education, learning and the introduction of new options, it is not possible for change to occur.

Anxiety can be triggered by a traumatic memory that is awakened when something similar to the original traumatic experience occurs. This is what is meant by "activation." An example is that if major traumas occurred at night, then just the onset of the night can evoke anxiety. Night time, for instance, is activating for abuse survivors who were sexually assaulted at night.

When anxiety begins there is no distinction between past and present. Once that distinction is clear to the body as well as to the mind, anxiety has more difficulty initiating. The applied touch protocols provided in this chapter interrupt the neuronal and sensory process of anxiety. Just the act of touching yourself with compassion and sending a message of safety on the sensory highway of your skin to your brain interrupts anxiety.

If you consistently interrupt anxiety, even if you do that mid-stream, it will eventually stop firing. Disturbing experience has a massive impact on neurology, much more so than positive events. It takes the consistent repetition of positive and calming experiences to turn down the high volume of negative, traumatic experience. Unfailing, loving devotion to self-care makes the crucial difference and brings the reward of erasing anxiety. Do not be discouraged. Even if you intervene after the onset of an anxious response and then backtrack later, you are still interrupting the pattern. Do not blame or criticize yourself. Keep moving forward.

The simple interventions that follow send signals to your problem solving brain centers to take charge and interrupt the pattern of anxiety. The more frequently you use the practices, the greater their potency. Your courage to heal mirrors to others that they can do this too. Just observing you unwinding from your anxious behavior will be inspirational and instructive. That possibility alone makes trying these strategies worth the experiment even if they do not make sense to you at first. Healing is as contagious as trauma.

Everyone has their own anxiety choreography. It is not the same dance for everyone. The applications below, therefore, refer to some of the most typical forms of anxiety. Find those that match your experience and use them each time you catch yourself on the road to anxiety. Apply your chosen self-care as soon as possible when you recognize that you are activated. Even if you have gone three-quarters or halfway down the activation highway before you remember to try self-care, you have not failed. As you pay attention you will start to catch the anxious onset sooner and sooner and eventually it will disappear completely.

Anxiety with Exhaustion

The coupling of anxiety with exhaustion is common. One leads to the other. Exhaustion itself will kindle anxiety. That is why the treatment of anxiety with exhaustion aims at adrenal repair. Exhaustion is also the kindling wood for the fiery explosions associated with head injuries. People with head injuries should therefore avoid fatigue and use rest as an antidote.

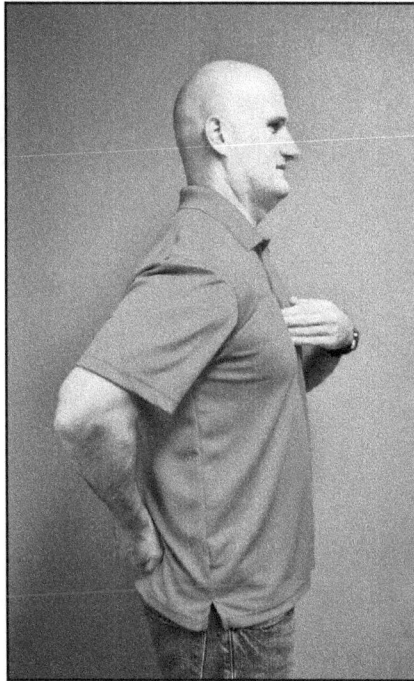

Figure 8.4

This is the Adrenal Tonifier. It helps repair the damages of over-adrenalization which inevitably lead to exhaustion. The illustration shows the holding of the top of the coccyx and the center of the chest which is identified as Middle 13.

Anxiety with Fear

Hold the right index finger and then the left index finger. You will feel a pulse from the finger coming into the hand that holds it. Follow this with holding #14 (under the ribs on the front of the body) with #23, which is directly behind #14. Hold these two sites first on the right side and then on the left side.

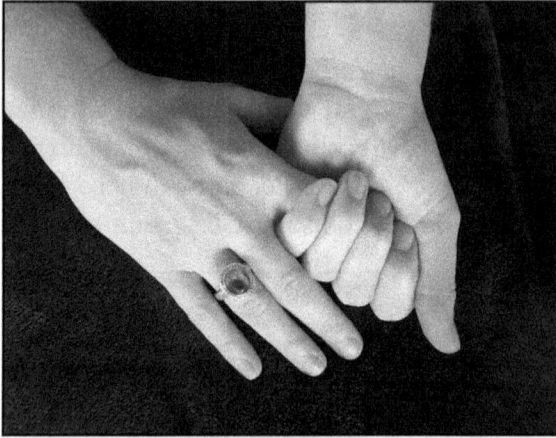

Figure 8.5

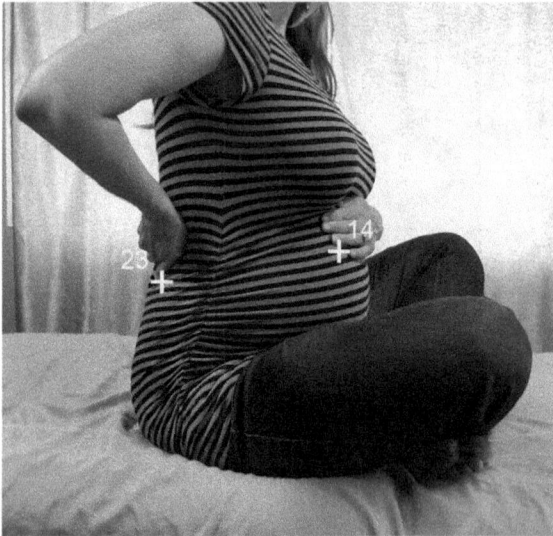

Figure 8.6

Anxiety with Obsessive Thinking

1. Hold the right thumb and then the left thumb.
2. Next hold both the right and the left #22 simultaneously.
The pulse from this position under your collarbones will rise up
into the fingertips you have selected to contact these sites.

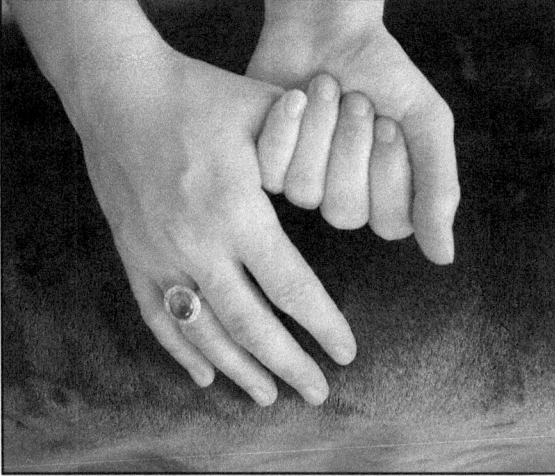

Figure 8.7

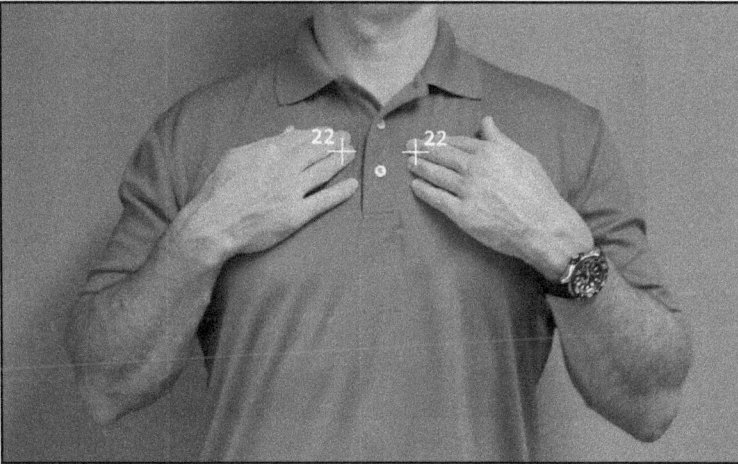

Figure 8.8

Anxiety with Racing Heartbeat

1. Hold the right little finger and then the left little finger.

2. Then identify the area between the little finger and the ring finger on the palm of your hand. Gently press into that area, first on the right side and then on the left side. You may use any finger or fingers to do this.

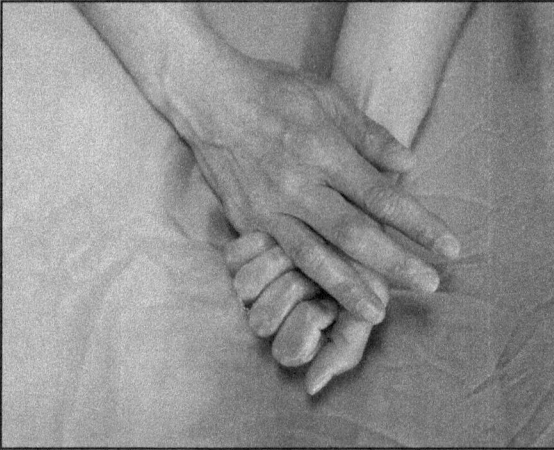

Figure 8.9

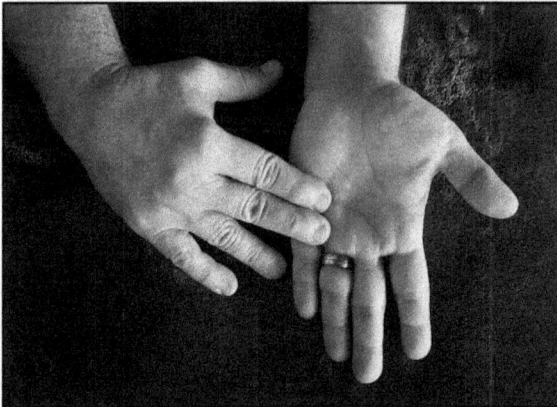

Figure 8.10

Anxety with Rage:

1. Hold the right middle finger and then the left middle finger.

2. Then hold #12 first on the right side and then on the left side. These can also be held simultaneously if that is comfortable.

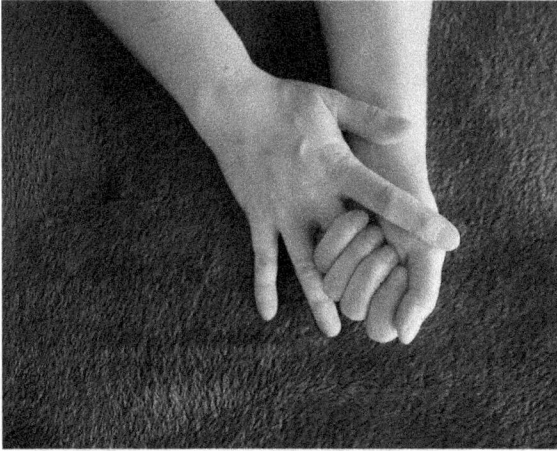

Figure 8.11

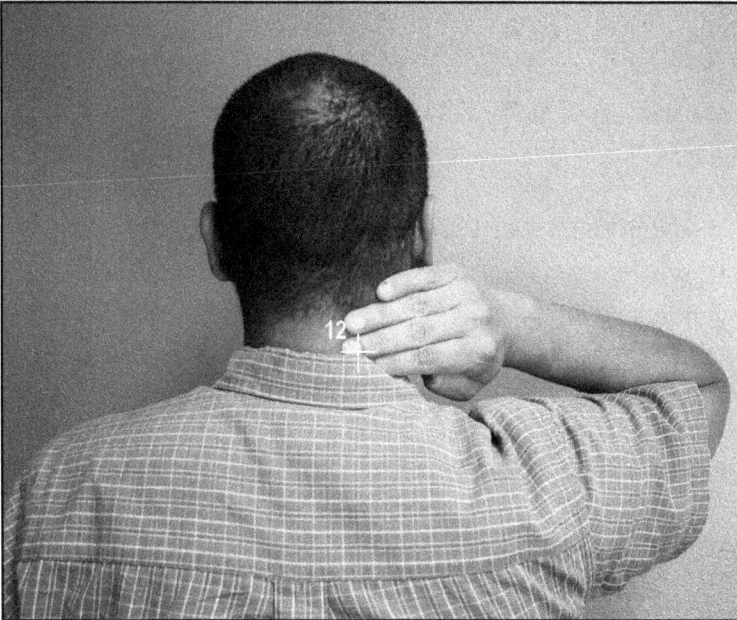

Figure 8.12

Anxiety with Trembling and Shaking

Hold #26 on one side and #24 on the opposite side, as illustrated. If this is uncomfortable simply hold the sites individually, one at a time.

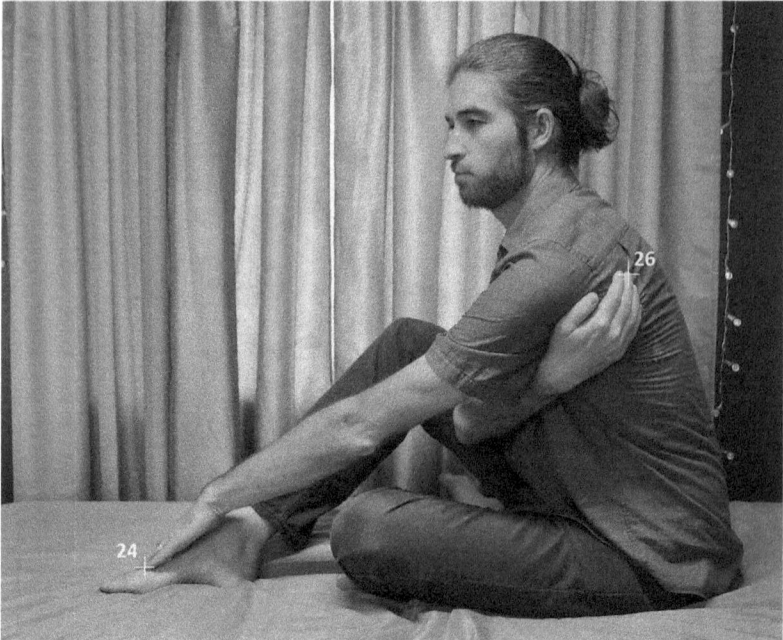

Figure 8.13

Attention, Awareness, Focus and Presence

Clearing the mind is the first step to clearing the body. An ancient adage is: "Where the mind goes, the body follows." This matches the neurological rule of thumb that says, "What fires together, wires together." This means that what we repeat we become. We do not want to repeat a confusion of ourselves with trauma. The sooner we can disengage that misconception, the better.

There are three simple steps you can take physiologically to initiate clarity, attention and focus. These are essential for growth and sustained healing. Focus always cuts through distress and chaos. These practices are also antidotes to disassociation, emotional numbing and hyperactivity.

#1: Hold the top or the crown of your head with your right hand and the center of your forehead with your left hand. The palms of your hands can rest fully in these positions or you can use your fingertips if you prefer. The center of the forehead position is known as Middle 20.

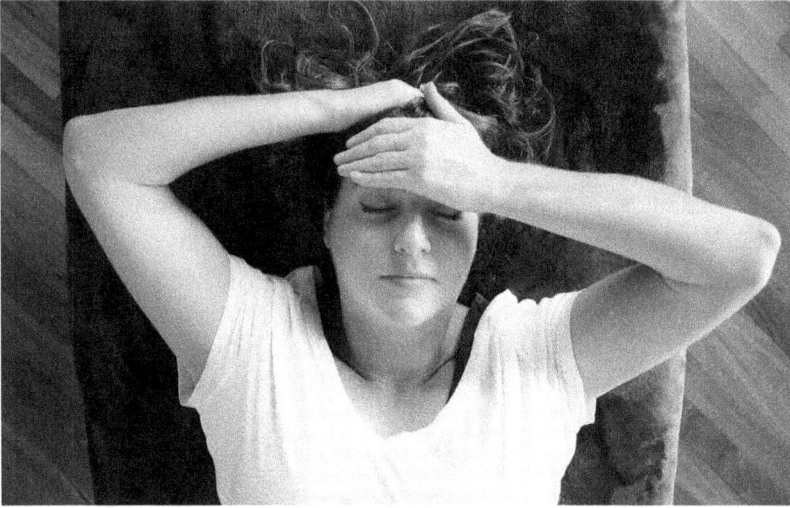

Figure 8.14

#2: Cross your arms in front of you so that your fingertips rest in the crevice that is at the bend of your elbow. These positions are #19 and if you look at the map of the sites you will see that they relate to setting boundaries. You are setting a boundary around your body to disconnect from the trauma fumes. You are clarifying that you are not available for the infection. You are unwilling to be contaminated. Learn more about boundaries further on. They are a central concept for us to embody.

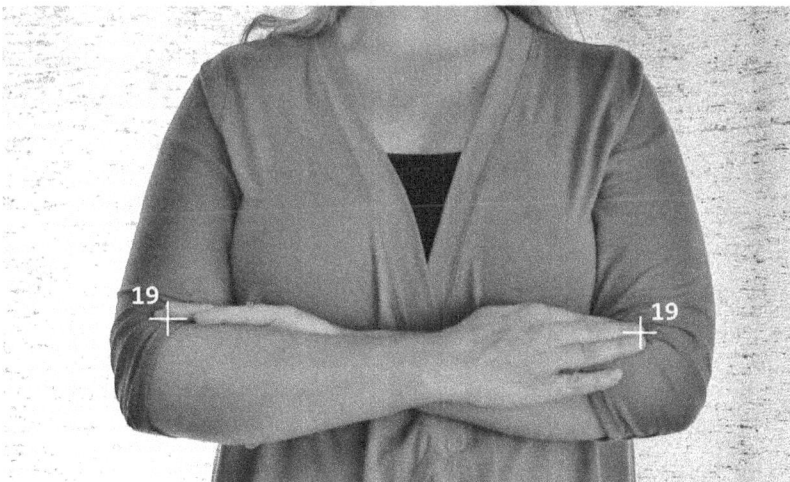

Figure 8.15

#3: Hold #17 on the left hand and then on the right hand. This small but amazing area helps your nervous system to quickly sort out distractions and discard them. This is perhaps the most discreet practice of all as your hands can rest comfortably on your lap or even behind your back as you do this. You can be standing or sitting. This simple action clears your mind and brings you into the present. You can also use Site #17 by itself to help you find clarity whenever you are overwhelmed or confused. It helps you sort out and determine priorities.

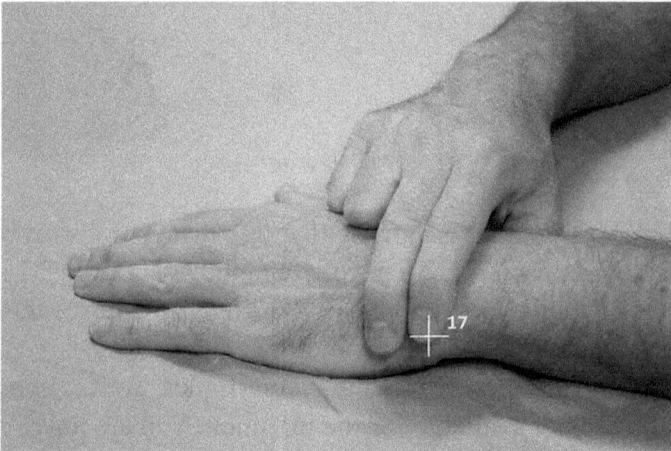

Figure 8.16

Attention Disorders

Attention Deficit Hyperactivity Disorders (ADHD) that may have been undetected prior to service and then exacerbated by combat are components of trauma when war comes home. The combination of forgetfulness, being jumpy and agitated, poor focus and scattered attention reap confusion and disorganization. To whatever degree the following practices are helpful, they are treasures!

Hold the same side #11 and #25. You can do this on the right side or the left side or both, in whatever order you select.

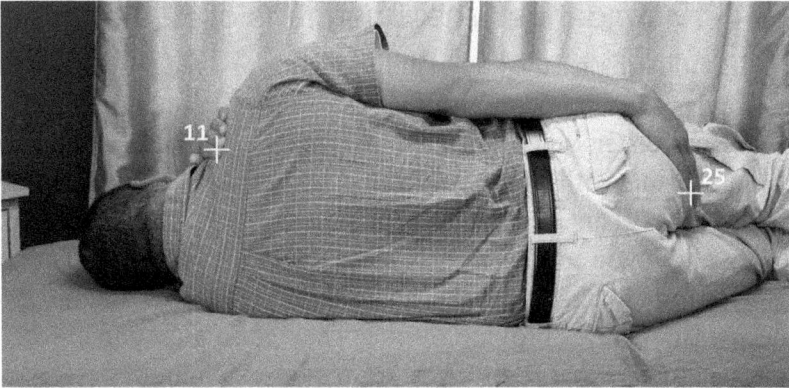

Figure 8.17

The first area that we introduced in this chapter, #1, is a helper for ADHD. Like holding #11 and #25, this simple gesture will still and calm both the mind and the body.

In the tradition that Mary Iino Burmeister transmitted to me there are hand postures called Inju that are super-efficient practices. The one that is probably used the most is called Palm Inju and it looks like your hands are in a prayer position. This Inju is a comprehensive way to reach a state that is referred to as "centered" or coming into mind-body alignment. Another word for this state is "congruence." It means you are "all together" or "at one with yourself." This state counteracts hyperactivity or scattered behavior. Corporate executives use centering to zero in on their goals and focus for success because it clears brain static.

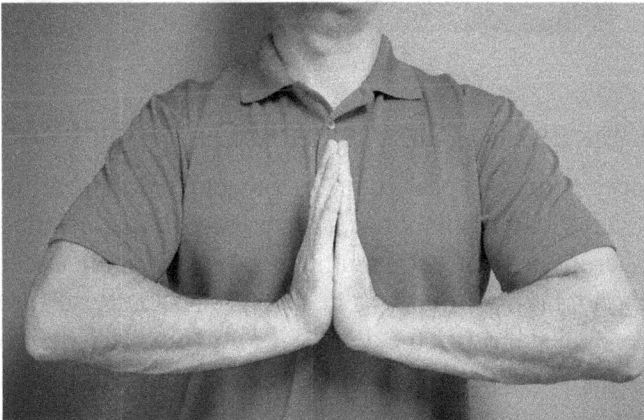

Figure 8.18

Boundaries: The Guaridans of Health

Boundaries are the key to individuation and the prevention of Secondary Traumatization. What is meant by boundaries? Mary Iino Burmeister, who translated the system of applied touch that I am sharing with you here, called boundaries "your personal bodyguard." This means that boundaries protect you from harm. They allow you to move away from danger, to say no when no is appropriate and necessary, and to honor your own health and needs. Boundaries provide respite. They erase guilt and enforce the sanctuaries that shelter you from over-extending.

To potentize your capacity to set boundaries and really mean it we employ High 19 which bears the title of Really Good Boundaries.

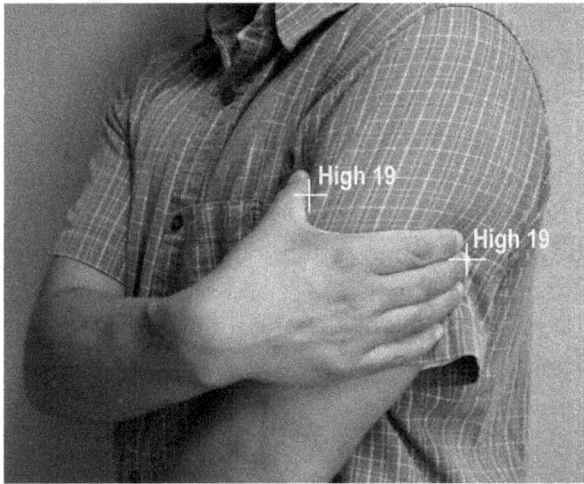

Figure 8.19

Depression, Despair and Disappointment

Depression, despair, disillusion and disappointment are threaded intricately into the war experience. In fact PTSD should be an acronym for Post-Traumatic Stress Despair except it is actually not "post;" it is present. This is especially so for family members who confront the depressive downloads in their present time living rooms and bedrooms. Because the returning service member has center stage and is the "identified patient," the family members who reel from what is unresolved push their own despair aside. This is especially true if there are children to protect. Family members almost always carry serious financial concerns that add to the mix of stressors. It is not surprising that despair and depression are undercurrents, if not major waterways, in the geography of war coming home.

The following treatments can shift neurochemistry just enough to allow smoother sailing. I have used them frequently in the writing of this book. They have allowed me to stop swirling in the vortex of trauma that accompanies this material. It is a palpable relief to find that the burdensome weight of pain is lifted just by sitting quietly holding areas of your body. The lightness descends and you are buoyed up and onward, as if someone put wind in your sails.

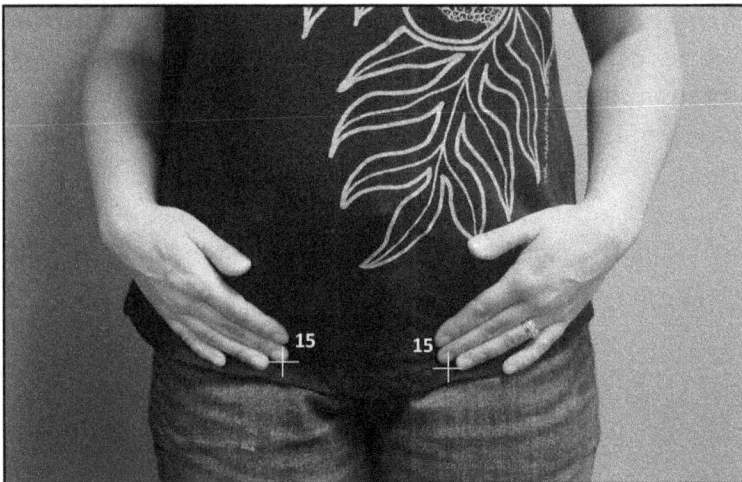

Figure 8.20

My teacher Mary called Site #15 the body's antidepressant. She also referred to it as "Wash Your Heart With Laughter." Site #15, along with the option of holding Site #15 with Site #2 that follows, both may require a private place for the application. These sites open you to a new world of possibilities that cuts through the density of despair.

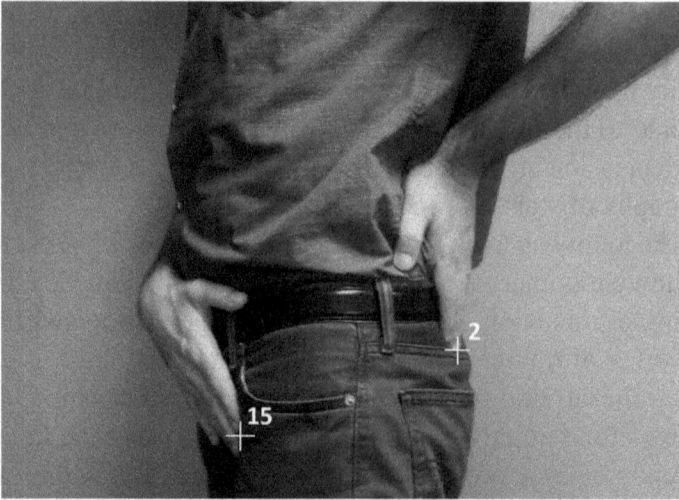

Figure 8.21

Sites #15 and #2 represent inspiration. Inspiration is what antidotes depression and despair. These sites also free any restrictions in the hips. Think of the parallel functions of hip liberation and inspiration. The two together spell the freedom to move in any direction. The felt sense of being able to access new options is what frees us from the trap of depression just as holding these two sites frees us from the restrictions of sciatica.

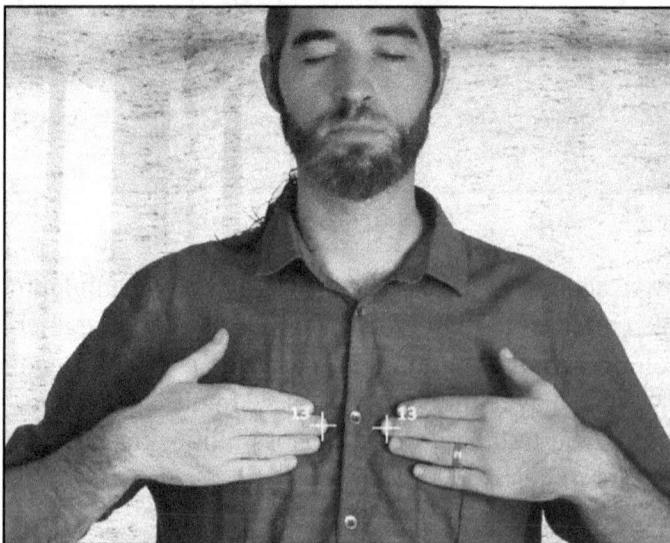

Figure 8.22

Holding the Right and Left 13 simultaneously lessens over-load. The feeling of there just being "too much" is often behind despair. Site #13 is considered to be the emotional center of the body. Like Site #17 this site stimulates an innate capacity to sort priorities and thereby erase overwhelm. This inherent, natural process can get buried under stress. I have used this site, along with all the others described here, throughout the writing of this book in order to differentiate from the mammoth nature of the topic of how war comes home and articulate what is of value.

Exhaustion and Fatigue

It is very difficult to maintain awareness, presence, clarity and boundaries when you are exhausted. Fatigue makes you vulnerable to Secondary Traumatization. It kindles neurological injuries. For quick relief from fatigue hold Site #18 at the base of the thumb. This will not only wake you up, it will also clear your head so that you can take positive action.

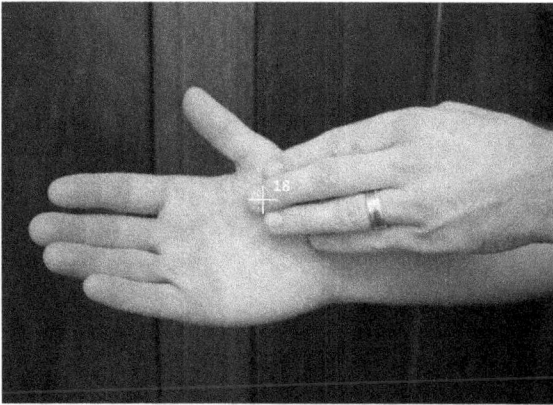

Figure 8.23

You can also use this Inju, which I call the Inju of the Physi-cian, to wake you up. This, like Figure 8.4 is an Adrenal Tonifier. You can use both applications for fatigue.

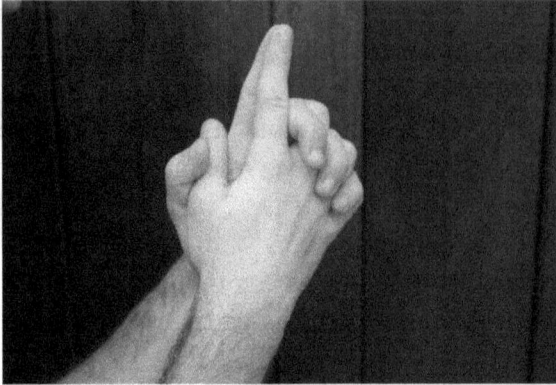

Figure 8.24

You can also excuse yourself for a quick rest and lie down holding #25. Five to ten minutes can be surprisingly regenerating. Site #25 is called Quiety Regenerating and is located at the base of the buttocks. Just slipping your hands onto the right and left 25 will result in a new you. This site could also be called Respite!

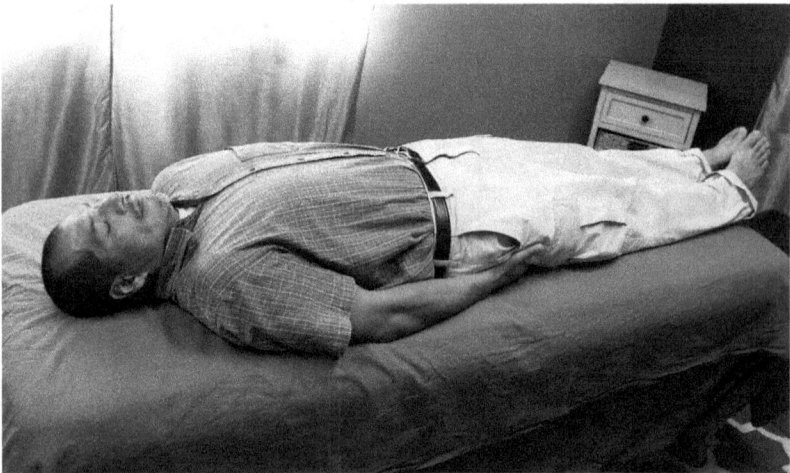

Figure 8.25

Insomnia, Nightmares, Restlessness and Sleep Disturbances

Good sleep is a natural healer. To support your capacity to rest and sleep well, use these applied touch practices at bedtime.

Hold the crown of the head and the base of the sternum. These sites are not numbered though the sternum position is considered the Middle #14.

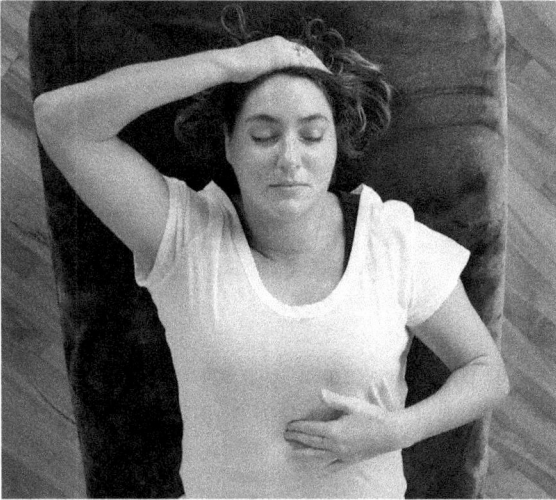

Figure 8.26

Hold both the right and left #14.

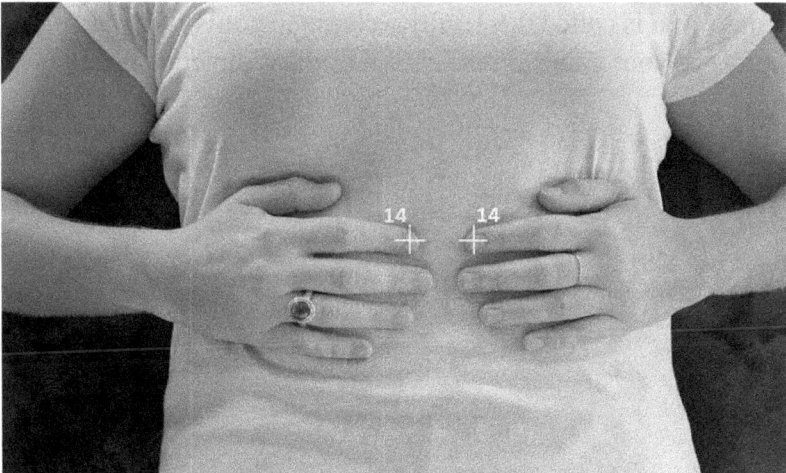

Figure 8.27

Hold #21 with the same side #22 on one side and then the other.

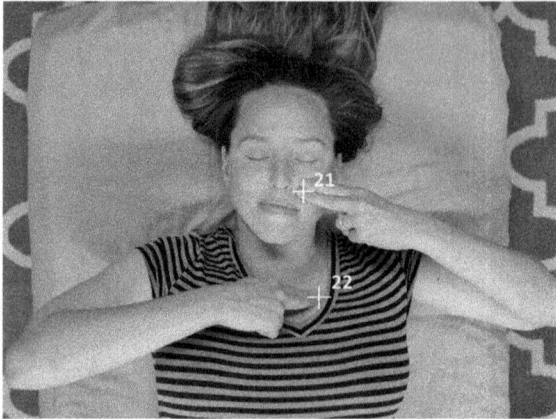

Figure 8.28

You can do these practices in a series or you can do any one of them individually. You can also do these practices in the order you prefer.

Panic

You can help a child who is panicked both by using the Palming the Calves intervention suggested earlier in the book, or by using what is called the Trinity Release that involves placing the palms of your hands on the crown of the recipient's head.

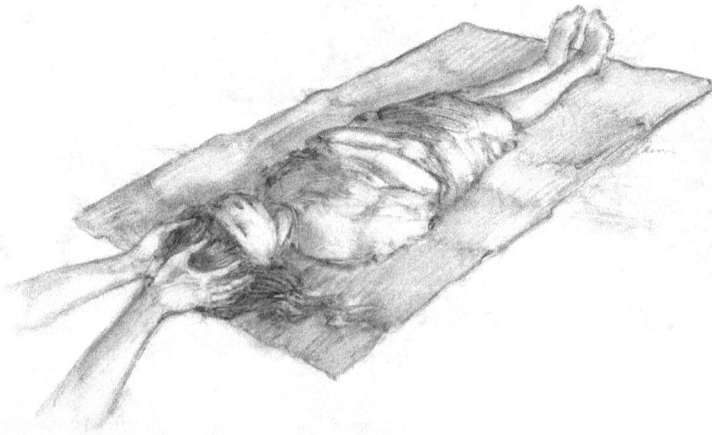

Figure 8.29

For an adult who is activated either by witnessing someone else's panic attack or because they are panicked, the following treatment restores calm and allows the nervous system to find its symmetry.

Virtually all the interventions in this section contribute to lessening panic. Because panic comes on suddenly and rarely announces itself in advance, the use of the hands and the fingers is quick relief, interrupting the panic cycle as readily as possible before it escalates.

Holding the little finger calms the blood so that heart rate slows down. Holding the ring finger awakens the awareness of how our behavior impacts others. It brings us into relationship and deepens the breath. Bringing the hands together into a prayer posture, as mentioned previously, draws forth a sense of center that prohibits panic.

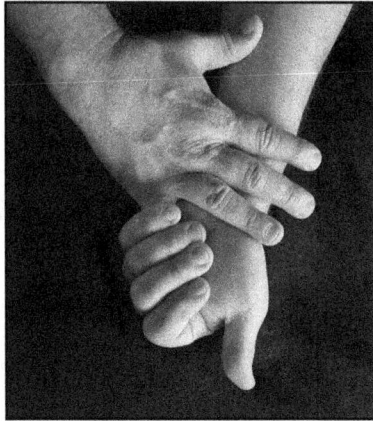

Figure 8.30

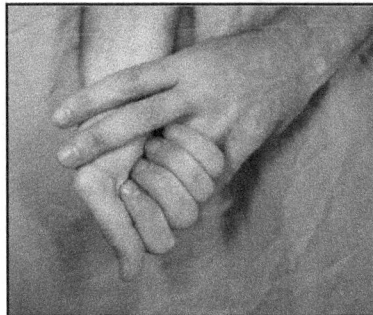

Figure 8.31

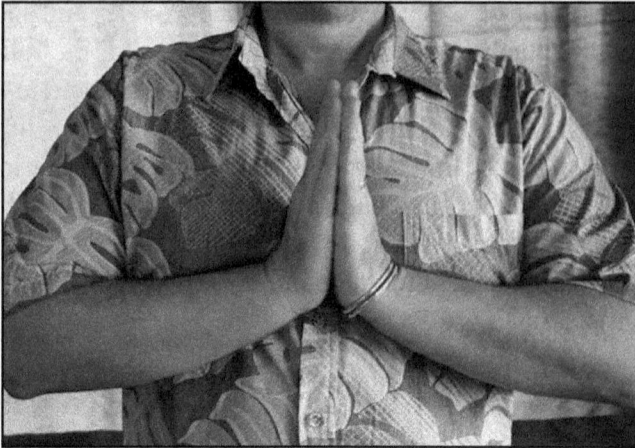

Figure 8.32

Palm or Prayer Inju, mentioned earlier, is a reliable way out of panic. In fact, this application will serve you any time you are disturbed, disoriented, disconnected or distracted. It brings you into the present with clarity.

Simply holding the index finger is an application that immediately speaks to the overstimulated nervous system and slows it down, bringing attention to the present. This is appropriate for any age. The index finger has been identified for multiple applications which is why I call it the finger of the physician.

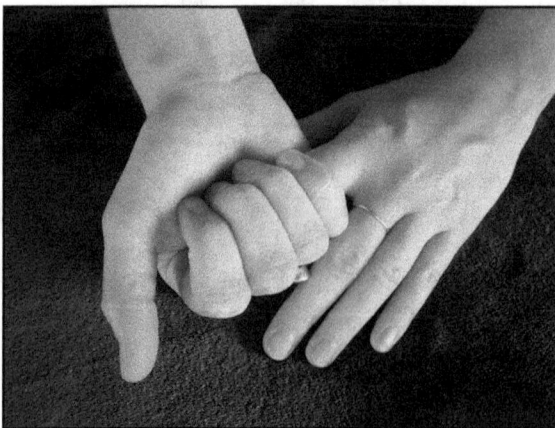

Figure 8.33

Sexuality and Self- Acceptance

Every family that I interviewed spoke candidly of how war steals healthy sexuality. The restoration of intimacy and safe sensuality is, I suggest, a component of an overall healing process. Patience and love are the remedies that can lead in that direction. To support these possibilities I recommend the treatment for self-acceptance that requires holding Sacred Site #26. There are a variety of ways to hold this site. The first resembles giving yourself a hug.

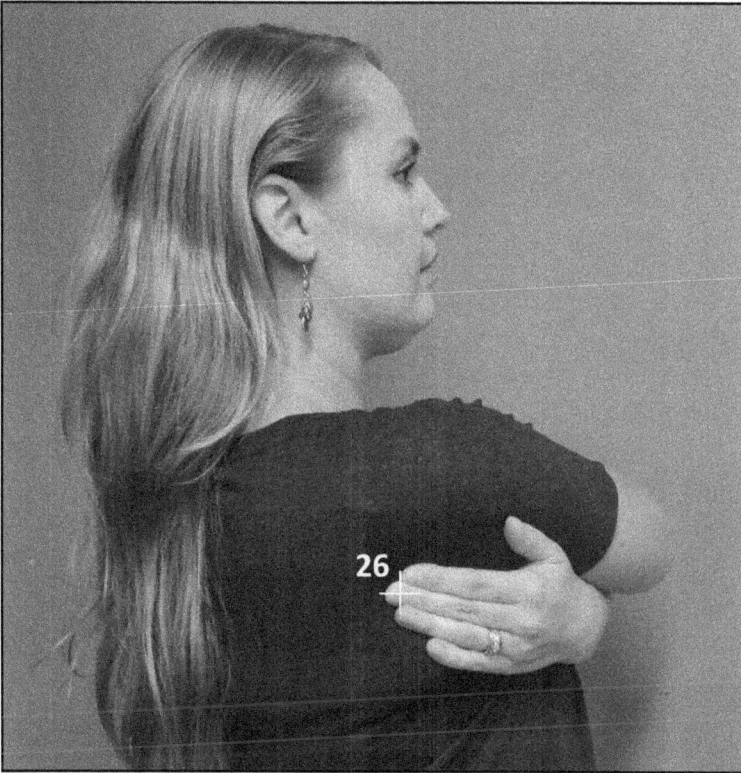

Figure 8.34

Another option is to hold Sacred Site #26 and on that same side place the palm of the thumb on the ring fingernail, forming an Inju or finger posture. This allows self-acceptance to merge with the release of grief.

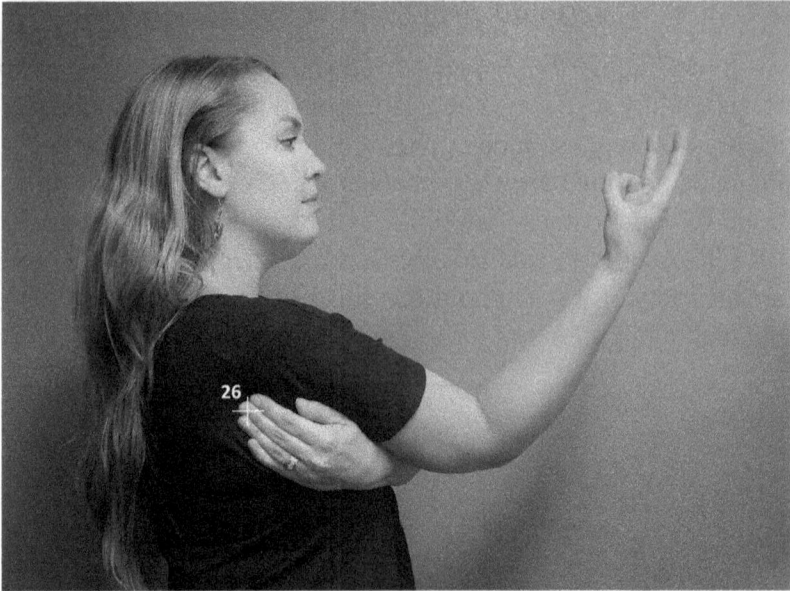

Figure 8.35

These applications are intended as an introduction to the possibilities of using applied touch in rituals of regeneration to invoke nervous system balance. More treatments for shock are available in my book *We Are All in Shock*[8] and for children in *New Frontiers in Sensory Integration*.[9] Workshops, courses, handbooks, videos and options for training can be found on my website.[10] I look forward to hearing about your responses to the use of these applications. You can add to your repertoire the holding of all of the fingers for the states of mind that are indicated in the illustration for them. Children enjoy knowing about these options and use them readily.

The TARA Approach and New Forums Press is committed to creating opportunities for the families of veterans to expand their self-healing capacities. Please contact us directly if you would like to create an opportunity for your community.

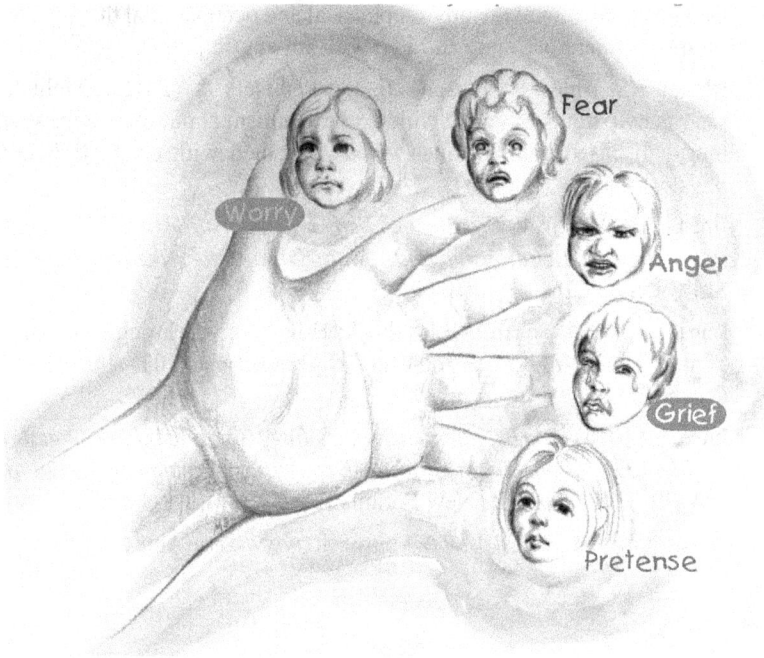

Chapter 8 Notes

1. If you would like to read or reference the published clinical results of research demonstrating the effectiveness of the TARA Approach's applied touch subtle energy medicine component in the treatment of stroke you will find it in the journal *Complementary Therapies in Medicine*, Vol. 18. February 2010; see also the following citations:

2. Hernandez, T.D., McFadden, K., Segal, A., Ivankovich, B.G., Gavito, C., Huerta, S. Effectrs of Jin Shin on Motor Function following Stroke (abstract). JINS 2007;13, Suppl S1. DOI:10.1017/S1355617707079969:http://journals.cambridge.org/action/displayIssue? Jid=INS&volumeId=13&issueId=S11;

3. Hernandez, T.D., McFadden, K., Segal, A., Ivankovich, B.G., Gavito, C., Huerta, S. Functional Improvement after Stroke: A Role for Complementary Medicine. *Journal of Neuropsychiarty Clin Neuroscience*. 2007; 19:213;4.   Hernandez, T.D., Ramsberger, G., Kurland, J., Hadler, B. *Functional Consequences of Jin Shin TARA Treatment after Stroke: A Preliminary Investigation.* Society for Acupuncture Research Abstracts. 2003; 43;

5. Mines, S., Morris, T., Persun, D. and Petersen, D., (2014). A randomized, blinded, controlled study to compare the efficacy of applied touch, physi-

cal and occupational therapy vs. physical and occupational therapy alone in the treatment of young children with autism (in press).

6. Erdman, R., Mines, S., Persun, D., and Petersen, D. (2015), Qualitative reports by parents of young children with autism about experiences with meridian based applied touch when combined with occupational and physical therapy (in press).

7. Mines, S. (2014) *New Frontiers in Sensory Integration: Limbic Stimulation, Authentic Relationship and a Multi-Disciplinary Treatment Design.* Stillwater, OK: New Forums Press.

8. Mines, S. (2003) We Are All In Shock: How Overwhelming Experiences Shatter You....And What You Can Do About It, pgs 103 - 140. NJ: The Career Press

9. Mines, S. (2014) *New Frontiers in Sensory Integration: Limbic Stimulation, Authentic Relationship and a Multi-Disciplinary Treatment Design*, pgs 75 – 99. Stillwater, OK: New Forums Press

10. Website for Dr. Mines' TARA Approach: www.Tara-Approach.org.

Chapter Nine

Networks of Care: Resources for the Families of Veterans

Think of this section as a compass. It points you towards available resources and how you can determine if you want to move in their direction. I also provide guidelines and cautions about outreach to protect you and your family.

Family members who feel discouraged by the lack of awareness in the civilian population and the antiquated bureaucracies of government agencies have another option. The independent non-profit organizations, many founded by service families, are on board to prevent the deepening scars of war. Whenever possible I have included these organizations.

Early intervention is so important that I want to shout out the words. The sooner effective resources are identified and used proactively, the less likely that the contagion of war becomes widespread. The ramifications of going without support and realistic, practical guidance are devastating. They are documented in the suffering of countless individuals as well as in collected data and even in literature. Reading novels like Toni Morrison's *Home* or *Carthage* by Joyce Carol Oates gives you a picture of how rampant and untreated moral wounds escalate into crime and destruction, reverberating through generations. Both books are based on real events.[1,2]

It is also true that healing does not have a time limit. Knowing that early intervention is essential does not mean that it is ever too late. The time to act to identify and harness networks of care is always NOW.

It is not possible to itemize all the available networks of care in any location, much less throughout the US and abroad. Rather than even attempting such a list, my purpose is to emphasize how to find and create networks of care and resources in a way that is focused, educated and self-advocating. My investigations have been restricted to the US and the UK for the purposes of this publication. I do not list websites as these are highly changeable. I emphasize references to stable, dependable organizations and publications.

Unfortunately there are individuals and organizations that exploit funding that is available for veterans and their families. Networking exposes us to this. Basic cautionary principles allow us to avoid being duped. Be cautious and educated when you search. You can easily vet the legitimacy of any organization by verifying their nonprofit status through Charity Navigator or the local Better Business Bureaus in the US, or equivalent agencies abroad. Evaluate reviews, speak to people directly and do not provide personal or financial information as legitimate services will never require it. You can, and should, cross-reference any site or organization by consulting with another trusted organization. Make sure all contact information is functional and that addresses are substantiated. Another inquiry is whether the organization actually uses its funding for veterans. According to the American Institute of Philanthropy many charities spend less than 60% of their budgets on bona fide charitable programs.[3] If at any time, any conversation or contact feels "not right", trust that feeling and move on. There are a multitude of options and a cornucopia of resources that will meet your needs and satisfy your quest. You never have to settle for anything other than what you truly want. Self-advocacy in all things is the bottom line!

In regard to resources for children, there are additional preparations that enhance the quality of your outreach. The more you know about your child, the more you can assess available networks of care and educational opportunities. There is a concept that is known as niche construction that I appreciate. This concept emphasizes attunement to the child with a focus on their gifts, and then matching resources to nourish those gifts. In this light, resources are seen as enhancements and investments in intelligence and potential, and not as corrective or as a response to a deficiency. The idea of niche construction evolved out of reframing special needs or disabilities, and seeing them as aspects of diversity rather than as disorders. This is similar to the development of the term "neurodiversity" as a way of framing neurological differences such as autism or sensory needs.

Using this prism to see how to select resources for children, we can not only choose programs, books, camps, educational options and services, we can also select the individuals who will most congruently match the needs of an individual child. Of course this same attitude applies to finding resources for adults. Children, however, need stewards or advocates who steer this process for them. Adults are the voices for children, and we are also their eyes in regard to selecting where they will go and who will be assigned their care when we are not there. To do this best we therefore need to consider:

1. Each child's developmental needs;
2. Whether or not the child has specific sensitivities, including sensory needs, that have to be honored in their environment; and
3. What are the child's special interests and gifts that would benefit from nourishment and cultivation?

At its best, networking erases feelings of isolation and fragmentation. The experience I had searching for others serving the families and children of veterans exemplifies this. I discovered Joy O'Neill, founder of the Service Children's Support Network in Britain this way. I connected with Joy as a result of a search on LinkedIn, a professional form of social media. Once I began a dialogue with Joy I recognized how aligned we were in our vision. This literally lifted me up. Realizing that we are never alone no matter how unique our experience shifts everything. It took some perseverance to find and communicate with Joy, but it was worth every moment. Connecting with others allows you take down one of the pillars of depression; the pillar which is the unproductive solitude of withdrawal and loneliness. Meeting Joy allowed me to feel part of an international team and motivated me to find more likeminded others. I knew they had to be out there!

I am certain that this quite limited offering of networks will breed a growing compilation. New Forums Press, publisher of this book, has made a commitment to cultivate such an expanding list on its website, where new contact information can be more easily adjusted digitally than is possible in a book. For that reason, what follows is suggestive and inviting rather than extensive. My purpose is to inspire you to gather up the patience and concentration it takes to do the outreach that will enhance and empower you and your family as you advocate for health and live the life you deserve to enjoy after war comes home.

I have organized the resources below into broad categories. I recommend reading about them from beginning to end so that you get a feeling for what is available. As you peruse the options you may feel an ah-ha moment when something that seems to have your name on it stands out. You will also have in your awareness other resources for families and individuals with need that are different from yours. Let me again remind you that this is a list intending to stimulate your curiosity and that it is not in any way comprehensive.

Resources for Children

In relation to young children, I have already mentioned Joy O'Neill throughout this book. I can recommend her organization in Britain, **Service Children Support Network**, wholeheartedly. Joy herself is both an early childhood education specialist and a military mother. She has written a children's book about mobility, entitled *Why Do We Have to Move?* She has also developed an online course to help educate about how childhood is impacted by the trauma that war brings home. Though Joy is based in the UK, her materials are appropriate no matter where you live. Contact her through her organization website for a copy of her children's book and to attend her online courses. Joy is available to consult with you about building networks for service children and bringing her model elsewhere.

I am confident in recommending an organization called **Zero to Three**. Check out their children's book *Sparrow Has Landed*, for instance, to experience directly the sensitivity with which they address deployment issues for the early years. This is a representation of their consistently excellent products. If you want to learn more about early development so that you can advocate specifically for your children and to assess what might fit best in their niche construction, then I recommend you inquire into the resources of **Zero to Three**. Their resources are universally applicable.

Chapters Three and Four of this book provide additional insights into what we need to do to protect our children and enhance their learning and healthy development. Chapter Four in particular refers to organizations created by service families to support their neurodiverse children, many of whom were diagnosed with autism. These include **ACT Today for Military Families**, **Autism Care**, and **American Military Families Autism Support Network**.

I also refer to Dr. Bruce Perry and his non-profit organization **The Child Trauma Academy** as a dependable resource.

The **TARA Approach for the Resolution of Shock and Trauma**, the system I developed, includes pediatric applications. These are provided in ongoing training programs throughout the US and in Scotland and Ireland. I have made several references to *New Frontiers in Sensory Integration*, my book with interventions for neurodiverse children. I have also written *The Dreaming Child* that provides general applied touch resources for children and is intended to be read by parents and children together.

Resources for Youth

A Backpack Journalist is a program designed specifically to encourage resilience through creative expression using writing, film-making, photo-journalism and related outlets. Programs are available throughout the US with special modules dedicated to military youth.

Camp Corral is a US based camp initiative that was developed specifically for youth whose military parent has been disabled, wounded or died in combat. The camps provide an outdoor, nature based experience of healing. Young people with similar struggles create an extended family for themselves, consisting of others who share their understanding of loss and recovery.

The Military Family Research Institute at Purdue University is a treasure. The staff has compiled, and keeps updating, lists of books and networking resources that they have vetted to assure their authenticity and value for military youth.

The National Military Family Association runs Operation Purple Camp in the US. This is a series of free, week-long summer camps around the country for the children of soldiers deployed overseas. They also provide **Operation Purple Camp for Children of Wounded Service Members**, incorporating additional mental health support into the camp activities. Check them out for help for spouses as well, including college scholarships.

Seeds of Hope Books are devoted to the experiences of adolescents who have a parent with PTSD or related mental health need. This publishing company invites and collects the writing of military youth who speak about what has happened to them in regard to deployment, loss and the emotional numbing of one or both parents. The founders of **Seeds of Hope** have direct and personal experience with the impact of current wars on youth and families. This is an important component in evaluating resources. Families and young people are sensitive to being viewed from within the experience rather than being seen by someone outside of it.

Resources for Families

The Foundation for Exceptional Warriors illustrates all the principles of proactive advocacy highlighted in this book. This private non-profit designs therapeutic recreational and sporting events for Special Forces veterans and their family members. Executive Director Ronny Sweger infuses this organization with his own healing experience and passion to reach out to exceptional warriors with opportunities for healthy reintegration.

Gov.UK has a number of branches dedicated to resources for military families in the UK in areas such as financial planning

(Money Force), mental health and wellbeing support and housing (Joint Services Housing Support).

Homes for Our Troops was developed by contractor John Gonsalves in the US. His heart went out to disabled veterans who needed living situations designed for their special needs. Today Mr. Gonsalves links with local businesses, other nonprofits and family members wherever he is called to serve. He supervises the construction of living environments that our wounded warriors can easily navigate and live in comfortably with their families.

Military One Source in the US is a comprehensive resource for families in all areas of the military.

Salute, Inc. is one of the remarkable organizations started by a service family to help other service families financially. Qualified recipients apply for funds to pay their mortgage, repair or purchase a car, or buy food. This is a US based resource initiated by a family that has been through financial hardship and is determined to protect other service families from experiencing isolation and abandonment when the going is rough.

Ed Tick and Kate Dahlstedt co-founded **Soldier's Heart** in 2006. The organization has become synonymous with the articulation of the soul wounds of war. Dr. Tick's remarkable books *War and the Soul* and *Warrior's Return* have drawn national attention to the moral suffering of war. Through retreats, workshops, publications, interviews and constant outreach Ed and Kate tirelessly advocate for the most authentic and timeless needs of veterans. As the organization has gained national attention **Soldier's Heart** has broadened its scope to include the families of veterans in retreats and special workshops. Kate Dahlstedt has spearheaded **Athena's Shield** to heighten awareness of the invisible wounds of female warriors and how we can tend to them.

In Scotland, compilations of resources for military families are available from **Veterans Assist Scotland**. Another related source in Scotland is **Armed Services Advice Project**. These are long standing agencies that are free to members of the military and their families. They both offer pamphlets and handbooks to help educate about trauma and family issues.

As you have read in this book, I have a direct knowledge of the networks developed and supported by **Veterans Families United (VFU)**. VFU reviews and publishes information about trustworthy agencies and resources on its website. It also periodically offers retreats and workshops for military couples, partners, individual family members, and families as a whole. Based in Oklahoma, where its activities generally occur, VFU is available worldwide as an information source about how war comes home and what we can do about it. Cynde Collins-Clark, LPC, who has learned directly how to advocate for a veteran with invisible wounds, responds to messages using her knowledge as the mother of a veteran. VFU also publishes and makes available an overview of PTSD from the veteran's perspective: *The Endless Journey Home: Post Traumatic Stress Disorder Symptoms and Resources*. This handbook is applicable to veterans and their families throughout the world.

Resources for Partners/Spouses

The **American Military Partner Association** is a nonprofit organization designed specifically to be of service to partners of veterans who are lesbian, gay, bisexual or transgender.

In the US, the **Department of Veterans Affairs** offers information and resources for the partners of veterans.

In the UK, the **Employers Network for Equality Inclusion (ENEI)** has devoted resources specifically to help the partners of veterans obtain employment. Along with this, ENEI provides workshops in other areas related to spousal issues like child care and special needs, information about benefits, housing, and debt management.

New Forums Press in the US, the publisher of this book, has made a commitment to provide e-books, blogs, networking directories and other resources at no charge to veterans and their families. They have published my handbook on emotional numbing, *Talking to Warriors*, which is a free download from their website. This e-book is directed to partners and other family members to assist them in coping with and responding to emotional numbing. *Talking to Warriors* and the other resources that New Forums Press provides can be accessed anywhere in the world and apply to military families worldwide.

The TARA Approach for the Resolution of Shock and Trauma, under the auspices of the Dom Project (a 501.c.3 nonprofit organization) sponsors and sustains outreach to the families of veterans and prepares resources for them, including resources designed specifically for children. Stephanie Mines, the author of this book, is the Program Director. If family members have an interest in participating in TARA Approach programs they can contact Dr. Mines directly through New Forums Press or the TARA Approach.

Local **Vet Centers** in the US provide counseling and workshops for veterans, their partners and families. There are 207 community based Vet Centers in all fifty states of the US, Puerto Rico, Guam and the District of Columbia. These are loosely affiliated with the Department of Veterans Affairs. Vet Centers are simultaneously independent and not subject to the restrictions and long waiting periods encountered at the VA. Vet Centers are staffed by local therapists and have a user-friendly and informal environment.

Veterans Families United (VFU), as previously mentioned, conducts and sponsors workshops for partners of veterans as well as seminars and retreats for partners. Visit the VFU website to be informed of these programs.

Visual Arts

The David Drakulich Memorial Art Foundation in the US is named for a veteran who used the expressive arts to communicate his experience and who gave his life during his service in Afghanistan. To honor his wisdom and lineage, his family created a foundation to support the use of the arts by veterans and their family members.

Integrating Therapy through the Arts (ITA) is an organization based in Chicago, Illinois that focuses on making creative arts, primarily visual and media arts, available to the families of veterans through its Operation Oak Tree. ITA has special programs specifically designed for children. ITA is a model of how the arts can be used for reintegration therapy to allow non-verbal processing when war comes home.

The Vet Art Project is a privately funded US organization that provides opportunities for veterans and their families to attend workshops at no charge to use creative media to address their war experience.

Writing

If spontaneous writing appeals to you as a method for jump-starting a writing practice, then you will benefit from reading **Natalie Goldberg's books** that are devoted to this technique. *Writing Down the Bones* is the primer.

The National Endowment for the Arts (NEA) in the US has created **Operation Homecoming**. You can download their *Operation Homecoming Workbook* from the NEA site to gain structure for your expressive writing practice. This is available to anyone, anywhere in the world.

The Veterans Writing Project in the US provides writing workshops for veterans and their family members. This nonprofit arose from the experience of veterans in Iraq and Afghanistan and is staffed by veterans and their family members.

Yoga

Many yoga centers have created their own version of yoga for veterans and their families. If these are not identified, taking any introduction to yoga or a class that is called restorative yoga is an excellent beginning. Restorative yoga focuses on relaxation. This is also sometimes called Yin Yoga. Yoga teachers tend to be highly receptive to ideas for classes. Partners of veterans can initiate a course specifically for military families to heighten the yoga options for their community. This holds true anywhere in the world that yoga is available.

If you would like to develop your own yoga practice at home using yoga for relaxation, the ***Relax and Renew* guidebook** by Judith Lasseter is a reliable source. There are a wide variety of yoga videos that can help support an at-home practice though there are benefits to taking periodic classes with an in-person instructor. If there is not a class specifically for veterans and their family members near you, local recreation centers frequently offer gentle beginning classes that can launch your use of yoga for de-stressing and as a ritual of regeneration.

The **Veterans Yoga Project** sponsors yoga classes for veterans and their family members throughout the US.

Yoga Warriors is an international organization that provides yoga classes and workshops specifically to address the wounds of war.

Summary

"If opportunity does not knock, build a door."
☐ Milton Berle

The essence of my message regarding developing resources to lessen the perseveration of the wounds of war is to be creative and proactive in seeking what is needed and if it does not exist, make it happen.. The families of veterans who have manifested structures in the US like **The Foundation for Excelptional Warriors, Salute, Inc.** or **Homes for Our Troops**, and Joy O'Neill's **Service Children's Support Network** in the UK, did so with grit, faith and determination. Now these models benefit others. Those who learn from war are the most likely teachers of peace. As Thich Nhat Hanh said, ***"Veterans and their families make peace with themselves and each other so they never have to use violence to resolve conflicts again."***

Chapter 9 Notes

1. Morrison, T. (2012) *Home.* New York: Vintage Books.

2. Oates, J.C. (2014) *Carthage.* New York: Harper Collins.

3. Glantz, A. (2010) *The War Comes Home: Washington's Battle against America's Veterans.* CA: University of California Press.

Chapter Ten

The REST House: Reintegration Environment and Service Transition

Origins of REST House

The REST House vision arises directly from the experience of how war comes home. It is a family centered and family inspired vision. For those veterans who have no family, it provides one for them. When Cynde Collins-Clark realized the magnitude of depression and despair her OIF (Operation Iraqi Freedom) veteran son Joe was carrying, she went into action to help him. Her quest became convoluted when the official avenues she explored turned into dead ends or even U turns that caused Joe to regress or worsened his condition. Cynde, like most civilians, assumed that a period of reorientation had been established by the military following a combat mission. She also assumed, as many civilians do, that VA care was "automatic." Neither assumption is accurate. There is minimal reorientation provided, particularly for Reservists, and all veterans must individually initiate application to receive VA benefits, which can be an overwhelming, confusing and lengthy process.

Cynde is herself a therapist and therefore she understands the terrain of trauma. She, unlike many other parents, was able to expand her search for support. She knew how and where to make inquiries in the local therapeutic community to which she belonged. Her investigations put her in contact with other families and she saw the universality of Joe's situation. I was someone

Cynde consulted for resources and when she told me her story I realized that it was my own. While I had decades of experience working with trauma, I had not directly encountered the needs of veterans or their family members. Perhaps I was even avoiding this issue as an escape from my own history.

Cynde's descriptions of how stranded she and other families were as they tried to get help for their wounded veterans confronted me with the memory of the landscape I inhabited as a child. War trauma invades the homes and bodies of veterans and their family members, and it seems that no one notices or cares. I certainly could not have articulated that analysis as a child, but that was what I experienced.

Cynde was unable to turn away from the needs of the other families she encountered just as she could not turn away from her son. She cultivated a vision for a way to provide the support, empowering resources, and keys to navigating the territory of re-entry that she was discovering. That vision was the seed of the REST House design but she was daunted at the prospect of manifesting it alone. When she shared it with me I found that I too could not turn away.

Out of our conversations came the formation of Veterans Families United (VFU), a nonprofit organization that then became the container for the REST House concept. VFU verifies networking information, and it also offers retreats and workshops in empowering healing systems. VFU's goals and the goals of this book are the same: to put into the hands of family members the tools, education, concepts and inspiration to reconfigure what happens when war comes home. VFU also publishes the booklet that Joe Collins, Cynde's son, wrote about his understanding of PTSD: *The Endless Journey Home.*[1]

What Is the REST House?

The REST House is a project designed to lay a strong foundation and serve as a model for transition from the traumatic experiences of war and readjustment. It is based on the premise that prevention and early intervention for service members who present with PTSD, polytraumas and related health problems after they return from active duty are the most effective. Our human capacity for innovation, creativity and resourcefulness are put to use for our veterans and their family members within the REST House design. The goal is to utilize holistic, person-centered paradigms to optimize the highest potential of all the individuals who are inevitably impacted when war comes home. The REST House design focuses first and foremost on the moral wounds of war and above all else provides inspiration, faith and community. Moral wounding goes hand-in-hand with survivor's guilt. It is the burden of wrongdoing that comes from both enacting and witnessing horrific acts of war and seeing team members killed when you were unable to protect them. Moral wounding is at the core of war trauma and combat shock.

The REST House is a time limited residential sanctuary that assures a supportive, mindful and therapeutic transitional structure as the readjustment from military priorities to a civilian lifestyle occurs. Basic amenities serve to alleviate stress for the family through:

1. Nutritional meals served to residents and to families when they come together for programs and therapeutic services;
2. Case management that tracks each veteran through the re-adjustment process, both individually and in the context of family dynamics;
3. Medical and dental care support and advocacy;
4. Development of a transition life plan;
5. Recreational activities for individuals and families;
6. Spiritual inspiration;
7. Evaluation; and
8. Documentation.

The REST House is designed to be an actual physical shelter established within a community. These residential settings serve both male and female veterans in a home-like environment. Depending on funding, the numbers of veterans in residence can vary. Applicants are assessed based on their need, resonance with the priorities of the REST House, space availability and capacity to follow protocols of behavior. The estimated stay is a minimum of one month and a maximum of one year.

Nutrition and Meals

Licensed nutritionists will develop meals and adjust them as needed for specific needs. The intention will be not only to serve quality food, but also to provide education about the role of nutrition in healing and recovery. Clients will participate in the planning, preparation, serving and clean up for all meals.

Case Management

A Lead Case Manager will be hired for each REST House and he or she will be supported by graduate interns in appropriate fields. A Treatment Coordinator will also be on staff. Each client will have their own individuated treatment plan.

Case management includes treatment and transition plans to determine:

1. Modalities suited to each client;
2. Family dynamics and family transition planning;
3. Financial counseling and planning;
4. Career counseling and planning;
5. Spiritual support;
6. Educational counseling and planning for career development;
7. Procuring benefits from appropriate agencies, including educational and rehabilitation services;
8. Implementation of benefits;
9. Overall transition to civilian life plan;
10. Development of ongoing self-care practices;
11. Stress management;
12. Stress relief programs;
13. Counseling and referrals for appropriate adjunctive services as needed; and a
14. Follow through plan.

The case manager will act as the "navigator" who will identify existing resources available in the community, supplement these with resources unique to the REST House, and create the continuity of care that is crucial for veterans and their families.

Treatment and Readjustment Training

Clients will have access to a broad spectrum of non-invasive healing modalities that are suited to their diverse needs. They will also have access to counseling as suits their particular situation, including interdenominational faith counseling. Family counseling will also be available for the family as a whole, for couples, and for individual family members including special services for children. These modalities will be holistic and somatic, such as energy medicine and energy psychology, yoga and related therapies, guided imagery, art therapy, movement therapy, mindfulness, meditation and prayer as well as other mind-body approaches that have demonstrated benefits for survivors of overwhelming experiences. The emphasis will be on modalities that can be replicated at home to foster the empowering follow through and sustainability that are the foundation of the REST House concept. The goal of REST House is not only to support readjustment and successful transition but also, whenever possible, to allow participants to grow and learn as a result of their opportunities to heal. Each REST House will provide the therapies that are available in their particular community and that are appropriate for the clients and families receiving services there.

REST House staff can support medical and dental care by accompanying clients to appointments and becoming patient advocates whenever necessary. The patient advocacy model will be an integral part of REST House as it supports learning empowerment skills whenever there are healthcare needs.

REST House will emphasize and maintain the development of a Transition Life Plan for each client. This may include vocational rehabilitation training with disability benefits when appropriate. When clients need support in envisioning new careers and new ways of being in the world, REST House staff will arrange appropriate team meetings or focus group dynamics that are based on self-inquiry and the conditions that allow individuals to genuinely quest within for new directions.

Recreation and Exercise

Recreation and exercise are essential components of each REST House design, incorporating families whenever possible. Depending on the geographical setting for the REST House, this will include a variety of outdoor sports. If possible clients can participate in gardening, growing food, and helping maintain the facility.

Children

Children are an integral part of the REST House programs. Pediatric therapists will be on staff. Whenever finances allow, each REST House will incorporate a "Family House" to allow residential options for family based activities. Staff members trained in helping children with trauma will develop children's programs. Play therapy, sand tray therapy, art and related expressive therapies will be available whenever possible to help children resolve Secondary Traumatization. Liaisons with school counselors and teachers will enhance the follow through for children and allow them to feel seen and heard as they manage the unique experiences of military children. Learning specialists will provide support for children whose traumatic experiences have impacted their learning development.

Interdenominational Spiritual Support

Space will be designated to encourage the spiritual aspect of healing. The term "moral injury" suggests that an essential component to a healing facility for combat veterans is to devote space and opportunity for spiritual growth and exploration. This may include an inter-spiritual chapel for meditation or prayer, a labyrinth or peace garden, and a small library for contemplative reading.

Each REST House facility will develop an interdenominational environment for spiritual support according to the needs of the clients.

Evaluation, Documentation and Publication

The evaluation and documentation process will be a significant aspect of each REST House. Statistics will be carefully maintained. Entrance and exit interviews will be conducted. Residents will be followed for a minimum of five years.

Statistics will also be maintained for the after-care process. Residents and family members will evaluate all aspects of the program and their evaluations will be carefully reviewed by staff on a regular basis.

Evaluation from staff will also be collected and reviewed regularly.

Qualitative studies will document the outcomes of the REST House paradigm and the publication of these will promote the REST House concept for increased implementation.

Summary Overview

REST House is intended to serve as a new model for prevention and early intervention for war related trauma and the impact of war on individuals, families, children and communities. The outcomes that can be predicted from the REST House vision are:

1. Reductions in mental health disabilities;
2. Lessening of medical needs for veterans and their family members;
3. Increased employment for veterans;
4. Enhanced quality of life for veterans and their families;
5. Resolution of addictive patterns;
6. Decreased incidence of domestic violence;
7. Decreased intergenerational traumatic repetition;
8. Enhanced contributions to society generally and to local communities where REST Houses exist;
9. Decreased exposure to abuse for children; and
10. Decreased divorce rates.

Finally, the research that results from the REST House experiment can propel us into a deeper understanding of the true cost of war and how to maximize options for healing the wounds of war for veterans and their families.

For every service member, there are a minimum of two significant family members who are directly affected. Emotional, financial, legal and relationship deterioration are but a few of the challenges that can domino into hopelessness for all involved. The REST House model is an early intervention vision that intends to de-escalate the inevitable contagion when war comes home. REST House is a viable healthcare model but it is also a model for humanity's sustainability. The nature of our current wars, including the increase in polytraumas and Traumatic Brain Injuries (TBI), along with exposures to toxic materials of unknown origins, has caused a skyrocketing of mental health, behavioral and medical problems. REST House is unique in that it presents a solution from within, based on the experiences of educated and attentive family members who are knowledgeable and thoughtful about what they have witnessed and endured.

This humane vision, once implemented, will gain increased substance and clarity. This refreshing optimistic structure is an investment in the future. We cannot afford to turn away from its promise.

Chapter 10 Note

1. Joe Collins, *The Endless Journey Home: Post Traumatic Stress Disorder Symptoms and Resources*, Oklahoma City, Veterans Families United ~ PO Box 14355, OKC, OK 73113 ~ www.VeteransFamiliesUnited.org.

Bibliography

Arango-Lasprilla, J.C., Ketchum, J.M., Dezfulian, T., et al (2008) 'Predictors of marital stability two years following traumatic brain injury.' *Brain Injury* 22(7-8): 565-574

Arnove, A. (2012) *Howard Zinn Speaks: Collected Speeches 1963 – 2009.* The Howard Zinn Revocable Trust. IL: Haymarket Books.

Bower, B. (2013) 'Heal Thy Neighbor: Mental health services recruit locals to help residents of poor and war-torn countries.' *Science News* 184: 22–26

Brock, R.N., Lettini, G. (2012) *Soul Repair: Recovering from Moral Injury after War.* Boston: Beacon Press.

Capps, R. (2011) *A Guide to Telling Your Own Story.* Veterans Writing Project. CreateSpace Independent Publishing Platform.

Capps, R. (2014) *Seriously Not All Right: Five Wars in Ten Years.* AZ: Schaffner Press.

Carey, N. (2012) *The Epigenetics Revolution: How Modern Biology is Rewriting our Understanding of Genetics, Disease, and Inheritance.* New York: Columbia University Press.

Carroll, A. (2006) *Operation Homecoming: Iraq, Afghanistan, and the Home Front, in the Words of US Troops and Their Families.* New York: Random House.

Castro, C.A., Kintzle, S., Hassan, A. (2014) *The State of the American Veteran; The Los Angeles County Veteran's Study.* USC Center for Innovation and Research on Veterans and Military Families. LA.

Chandra, A., et al. (2010) 'Children on the Homefront: The Experience of Children from Military Families.' *Pediatrics* Jan; 125: 16-25

Cozolino, L. (2006) *The Neuroscience of Human Relationships: Attachment and the Developing Brain.* New York: Norton.

Davidson, A.C., Mellor, DJ. (2001) 'The adjustment of Australian Vietnam Veterans: Is there evidence for the transmission of the effects of war-related trauma.' *Australian-New Zealand Journal of Psychiatry* Jun; 35(3) 345-351.

De Burgh, H.T., et al (2011) 'The impact of deployment to Iraq and Afghanistan on families of military personnel.' *International Review of Psychiatry* April; 23: 192-200

DiPietro, J.A. (2004) 'The Role of Prenatal Maternal Stress in Child Development.' *American Psychological Society*; 13(2): 71-74.

DiPietro, J.A. (2013) 'Fetal exposures to excessive stress hormones in the womb lead to adult mood disorders.' *Science Daily* April 7.

Doidge, N. (2007) *The Brian that Changes Itself: Stories of Personal Triumph from the Frontiers of Brain Science*. New York: Viking Penguin.

Dossy, L. (1993) *Healing Words: The Power of Prayer and the Practice of Medicine*. New York: Harper Collins

Eres, R., Decety, J., Winifred, R.L., Molenberghs, P. (2015) 'Individual differences in local gray matter density are associated with differences in affective and cognitive empathy.' *NeuroImage* Aug 15; 117: 305-310

Fegert, J.M., Ziegenhain, U. (2009) 'Early intervention: Bridging the gap between practice and academia.' *Child and Adult Psychiatry and Mental Health*; 3:23

Flynn, A. (2013) *Wife and War: The Memoir*. Rhode Island, USA. www.wifeandwar.wordpress.com

Francis, R.C. (2011) *How Environment Shapes Our Genes*. New York: Norton.

Galovski, T., Lyons, J.A. (2004) 'Psychological sequelae of combat violence: A review of the impact of PTSD on the veteran's family and possible interventions.' *Aggression and Violent Behavior* 9: 477-501.

Gilreath, T.D., Wrabel, S.L., Sullivan, K.S., et al (2015) 'Suicidality among military-connected adolescents in California schools.' *European Child and Adult Psychiatry* March.

Glantz, A. (2010) *The War Comes Home: Washington's Battle against America's Veterans*. CA: University of California Press.

Gopnik, A., Meltzoff, A.N., Kuhl, P.K. (1999) *The Scientist in the Crib: What Early Learning Tells Us About The Mind*. USA: William Morris & Co.

Gopnik, A. (2009) *The Philosophical Baby: What Children's Minds Tell Us About Truth, Love, and the Meaning Of Life*. New York: Farrar, Straus & Giroux.

Gregory, G.H. (2010) 'Wartime Military Deployment and Increased Pediatric Mental and Behavioral Health Complaints.' *Pediatrics* Nov; 126(6): 1058-1066

Hernandez, T.D., McFadden, K., Segal, A., Ivankovich, B.G., Gavito, C., Huerta, S. (2007) 'Effectors of Jin Shin on Motor Function following Stroke (abstract).' *Journal of the International Neuropsychological Society*; 13, Suppl S1.

Hernandez, T.D., McFadden, K., Segal, A., Ivankovich, B.G., Gavito, C., Huerta, S. (2007) 'Functional Improvement after Stroke: A Role for

Complementary Medicine.' *Journal of Neuropsychiatry and Clinical Neuroscience*; 19:213

Hernandez, T.D., Ramsberger, G., Kurland, J., Hadler, B. (2003) 'Functional Consequences of Jin Shin TARA Treatment after Stroke: A Preliminary Investigation.' *Society for Acupuncture Research Abstracts*. 2003:43

Hildebrand, L. (2014). Taken from an interview with Wil S. Hylton, '*The Unbreakable Laura Hildebrand'* in the New York Times, Sunday Magazine, Dec. 18th; pg MM36

Hoge, C.W. (2010) *Once a Warrior, Always a Warrior: Navigating the Transition from Combat to Home, Including Combat Stress, PTSD, and MTBI.* Guilford, CT: Globe Pequot Press.

Izzo, E., & Miller, V.C., (2010). *Second - Hand Shock: Surviving & Overcoming Vicarious Trauma.* Scottsdale, AZ: HCI Press.

Jones, A. (2013) *They Were Soldiers: How the Wounded Return from America's Wars –The Untold Story.* Chicago: Haymarket Books.

Jonikas, J.A., et al (2011) 'Improving Propensity for Patient Self-Advocacy Through Wellness Recovery Action Planning: Results of a Randomized Controlled Trial.' *Community Mental Health Journal* 2013 Jun; 49(3) 260-269

Kandel, E.R. (2006) *In Search of Memory: The Emergence of a New Science of Mind.* USA: W.W. Norton & Co.

Karshad, T.B., et al (2006) 'Anehedonia and Emotional Numbing in Combat Veterans with PTSD.' *Behavioral Research and Therapy* 44: 457 - 467

Klienman, A. (1988) *Social Origins of Disease and Distress: Depression, Neurasthenia and Pain in Modern China.* Yale University Press.

Klienman, A. (1988) *The Illness Naratives: Suffering, Healing, and the Human Condition.* USA: Basic Books Inc.

Kruetzer, J.S., et al (2007) 'Marital stability after brain injury: an investigation and analysis.' *NeuroRehabilitation* 22(1), 53-59.

Mathieu, F. (2012) *The Compassion Fatigue Workbook: Creating Tools for Transforming Compassion Fatigue and Vicarious Traumatization.* New York: Rutledge.

Max-Plank-Gesselschaft (2012) 'Childhood trauma leaves mark on DNA of some victims: Gene-environment interaction causes lifelong dysregulation of stress hormones.' *Science Daily*; Dec.

Mc Fadden, K.L., Healy, K.M., Detterman, M.L., Kaye, J.J., Ito, T.A., Hernandez, T.D. (2011) 'Acupressure as a Non – Pharmacological Intervention for Traumatic Brain Injury.' *Journal of Neurotrauma* Jan; 28(1):21-34

Milliken, C. S., et al (2007) 'Longitudinal Assessment of Mental Health Problems among Active and Reserve Component Soldiers returning from the Iraq War.' *Journal of the American Medical Association.* Nov 14; 298(18):2141 – 2148.

Mines, S. (2007) 'Domestic Violence Within Military Families.' *Encyclopedia of Domestic Violence*, NY, Routledge; 487-492.

Mines, S. (2014) *New Frontiers in Sensory Integration: Limbic Stimulation, Authentic Relationship and a Multi-Disciplinary Treatment Design.* OK: New Forums Press.

Mines, S. (1987) 'That Feeling of Not Being Seen as a Whole: Holistic Therapy and People with Disabilities.' *Dissertations International.* 48:6

Mines, S. (2003) *We Are All in Shock: How Overwhelming Experience Shatters You... And What You Can Do About It.* NJ: The Career Press.

Monson, C.M, Snyder, D.K (2012) *Couple Based Interventions for Military and Veteran Families: A Practitioner's Guide.* New York: Guilford.

Morris, D.J. (2015) *The Evil Hours: A Biography of Post-Traumatic Disorder.* New York: Houghton Mifflin Harcourt

Morrison, T. (2012) *Home.* New York: Random House.

Newberg, A., D'Aquili, E., Rause, V. (2001) *Why God Won't Go Away: Brain Science and the Biology of Belief.* New York: Random House.

Nicolson, G.L., Berns, P., Gan, R., Haier, J. (2005) 'Chronic Mycoplasmal Infections in Gulf War Veterans' Children and Autism patients.' *Medical Veritas* 2: 383 – 387

Oates, J.C. (2014) *Carthage.* New York: Harper Collins.

Parks, R.L., Reed, G.J. (1994) *Quiet Strength: The Faith, the Hope, and the Heart of a Woman who changed the Nation.* MI: Zondervan Publishing House.

Perry, M.P., Szalavitz, M. (2010) *Born for Love: Why Empathy is Essential – and Endangered.* New York: Harper.

Perry, M.P., Szalavitz, M. (2006) *The Boy Who Was Raised As A Dog: And Other Stories from a Child Psychiatrist's Notebook: What Traumatized Children Can Teach Us About Loss, Love, and Healing.* PA: Basic Books.

Purnell, C. (2010) 'Childhood Trauma and Adult Attachment.' *Healthcare Counseling and Psychotherapy.* April; 10: 2.

Ray, S.L., Vanstone, M. (2009) 'Impact of PTSD and Emotional Numbing on Veterans' Family Relationships.' *Nursing Studies.* June; 44: 6, 838 – 847.

Riabe, F.J., & Spengler, D. (2013) 'Epigenetics Risk Factors in PTSD and Depression.' *Frontiers in Psychiatry*, Aug7; 4: 80

Richardson, A., et al. (2011) 'Effects of Soldiers' Deployment on Children's Academic Performance and Behavioral Health.' Santa Monica, CA: RAND Corporation, 2011. http://www.rand.org/pubs/monographs/MG1095.

Rogers, C.R. (1980) *A Way of Being.* 142-143. New York: Houghton Mifflin.

Rohr, Fr R. (2008) To Be Awake is to Live in the Present. *Collection of Homolies 2008. CD,* MP3 Audio player.

Rosenheck, R., Fontana, A. (1998) 'Transgenerational effects of abusive violence on the children of Vietnam combat veterans.' *Journal of Traumatic Stress* Oct; 11(4):731-742.

Ruscio, A.M., et al. (2002) 'Male War Zone Veterans' Perceived Relationship with their Children: The Importance of Emotional Numbing.' *Journal of Traumatic Stress* Oct; 15 (5) 351-357.

Rychnnowsky, J. (2006) 'Screening for postpartum depression in military women with the Postpartum Depression Screening Scale.' *Military Medicine* Nov; 171 (11): 1100 - 4

Schore, A.N. (1994) *Affect Regulation and the Origin of the Self: The Neurobiology of Emotional Development.* New Jersey: Laurence Erlbaum Associates Inc.

Schore, A.N. (2001) 'Effects of a Secure Attachment Relationship on Right Brain Development, Affect Regulation, and Infant Mental Health.' *Infant Mental Health Journal*; 22(1-2) 7-66.

Schuengel, C. et al. (2009) 'Children with disrupted attachment histories: Interventions and psychophysiological indices of effects.' *Child and Adult Psychiatry and Mental Health*; 3:26

Schultz, H., Chandrasekaran, R. (2014) *For Love Of Country: What Our Veterans Can Teach Us About Citizenship, Heroism, and Sacrifice.* USA: Knopf.

Shepherd, B. (2000) *A War Of Nerves: Soldiers and Psychiatrist, 1914 - 1994.* UK: Jonathon Cape.

Sherman, M.D. (2008) *PTSD and its Impact on the Family: Mental Health Facts for Families.* Oklahoma City Veterans Affairs Medical Center.

Sherman, N. (2015) *Afterwar: Healing the Moral Wounds of Our Soldiers.* New York: Oxford University Press

Snyder, D., Monson, C. (2012) *Couple- Based Interventions for Military and Veteran Families: A Practitioner's Guide.* New York: Guildford.

Sogomonyan, F., Cooper, J.L. (2010) *Trauma Faced by Children of Military Families: What every Policymaker Should Know.* Columbia University Academia Commons

Thorpe, H. (2014) *Soldier Girls: The Battles of Three Women at Home and at War.* New York: Scribner

Tronick, E. (2007) *The Neurobehavioral and Social-Emotional Development of Infants and Children.* New York: W.W. Norton & Co.

Van der Kolk, B. (2014) *The Body Keeps the Score: Brain, Mind, and Body in the Healing of Trauma.* NY: Viking Penguin.

Williams, K. (2014) *Plenty of Time When We Get Home: Love and Recovery in the Aftermath of War*. New York: W.W Norton & Co.

Yehuda, R. (2007) 'Differentiating biological correlates of risk, PTSD, and resilience following trauma exposure.' *Journal of Traumatic Stress* 20(4); 435-437.

Yehuda, R., Bierer, M.L. (2009) 'The relevance of epigenetics to PTSD: Implications for the DSM-V.' *Journal of Traumatic Stress* 22(5); 427-434.

Yehuda, R., Cai, G., Golier, J.A., et al., (2009). 'Gene expression patterns associated with PTSD following exposure to World Trade Center attacks.' *Journal of Biological Psychiatry* 66(7): 708-711.

Yehuda, R., Daskalskis, N.P., Lehrner, A., et al. (2014). 'Influences of maternal and paternal PTSD on epigenetic regulation of glucocorticoid receptor gene in Holocaust survivor offspring.' *American Journal of Psychiatry* 171(8), 872-880.

Yehuda, R., et al. (2005) 'Transgenerational effects of PTSD in babies of mothers exposed to World Trade Center attacks during pregnancy.' *Journal of Clinical Endocrinology and Metabolism* 90(7): 4115-118.

Index

A

ACT Today for Military Families, 145
Adrenal Tonifier, 119
adrenaline, 28
advocacy, 15, 49
American Institute of Philanthropy, 142
American Military Families Autism Support Network, 145
American Military Partner Association, 148
anxiety, 118
aphasia, 110
applied touch, 61
Armed Services Advice Project, 147
art and related expressive therapies, 158
art therapy, 157
Athena's Shield, 147
attachment, 8, 35
attention, 124
Attention Deficit Hyperactivity Disorder (ADHD), 126
autism, 38, 56, 110
Autism Care, 145

B

Backpast Journalist, A, 145
bearing witness, 27, 90, 94
Beck, Lucille, 73
Bessel van der Kolk, 6
bioelectricity, 111
boundaries, 125, 128
boundary, 125
Burmeister, Mary Iino, 117, 127

C

Camp Corral, 145
Capps, Ron, 87
caregivers, 10
caregiving, 10

caregiving stewards, 10-11
Carl Rogers, 27
Carroll, Andrew, 101
centering, 91
Charity Navigator, 142
Child Trauma Academy, The, 64, 145
children of war, 53, 63, 104
clarity, 124
closed head injury, 70
Collins, Joe, 154
combat shock, 19
cortisol, 27

D

Dahlstedt, Kate, 147
David Drakulich Memorial Art Foundation, The, 149
decondition habituated behaviors, 110
Department of Defense, 72
depression, 24, 38
despair, 128
differentiation, 29
disassociation, 124
divorce rates, 74
DNA, 23
Dreaming Child, The, 145

E

early detection, 71
early intervention, 141
emotional numbing, 9, 38-39, 124
empathy, 11, 27
Employers Network for Equality Inclusion, 148
Endless Journey Home: Post Traumatic Stress Disorder Symptoms and Resources, The, 148, 154
epigenetics, xvii, 3-6
epinephrine, 28

About the Author

Dr. Stephanie Mines understands shock from every conceivable perspective. Her stories of personal transformation have led many to set out on a committed journey of healing. Her blend of Western and Eastern modalities offers the best of both paradigms. She is devoted to ending the lineage of shock and trauma for individuals and the world.

Dr. Mines is on the Board of Directors of Veterans Families United. Her experiences of how war came home to her family shaped her decision to study neuropsychology and to advocate for the children and families of veterans.

Dr. Mines teaches in the US and internationally. She is the founder of the TARA Approach for the Resolution of Shock and Trauma. TARA is an acronym for Tools for Awakening Resources and Awareness. She writes in several genres, conducts research, enjoys the natural world and her family, particularly her grandchildren Simone and Sophia.

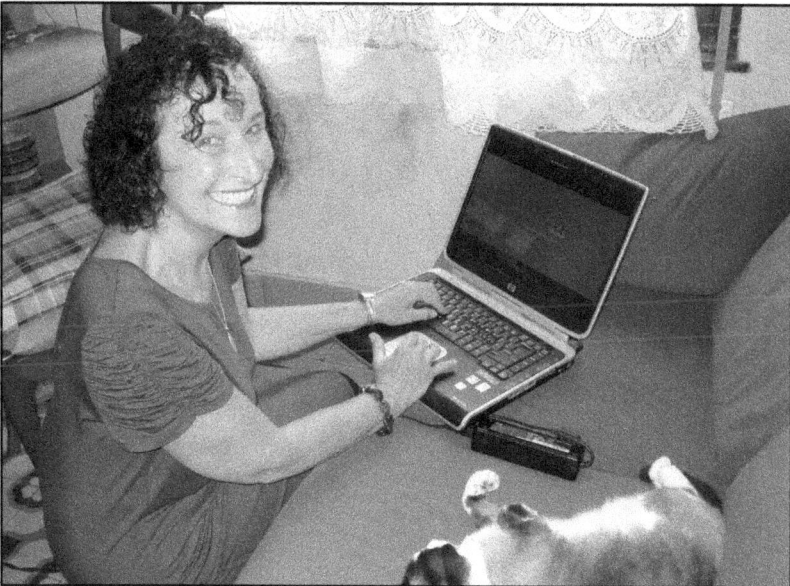

www.ingramcontent.com/pod-product-compliance
Lightning Source LLC
Chambersburg PA
CBHW071744270326
41928CB00013B/2789